Patients and Doctors

Patients and Doctors

Life-Changing Stories
from Primary Care

Edited by

Jeffrey M. Borkan, M.D.

Shmuel Reis, M.D.

Jack H. Medalie, M.D.

Dov Steinmetz, M.D.

THE UNIVERSITY OF WISCONSIN PRESS

The University of Wisconsin Press
2537 Daniels Street
Madison, Wisconsin 53718

3 Henrietta Street
London WC2E 8LU, England

2   4   5   3   1

Printed in the United States of America

Library of Congress Cataloging-in-publication Data

Patients and doctors: life-changing stories from primary care /
edited by Jeffrey M. Borkan . . . [et al.].
238 pp.   cm.
ISBN 0-299-16340-7 (cloth: alk. paper)
1. Physician and patient Anecdotes.   2. Primary care (Medicine)
Anecdotes.   I. Borkan, Jeffrey M.   II. Title: Life-changing stories
from primary care.
[DNLM: 1. Primary Health Care Personal Narratives.   2. Episode of
Care Personal Narratives.   W 84.6 P2982 1999]
R727.3.P39   1999
610.69'6—dc21   99-19758
DNLM/DLC
for Library of Congress

Contents

Foreword *George L. Engel* ix
Prologue *Arthur Kleinman* xi
Acknowledgments xiii
Introduction: Storytelling in Medicine
Jeffrey M. Borkan and William L. Miller 3

Chapter 1. Beyond the Call of Duty

Reflections *Robin Hull* 15

A Stormy Case of Appendicitis *C. J. Albert Rutulunyie* 20

The Cardiac Event, the Doctor, and the Wife *Shmuel Reis* 25

The Kiss of Life *Ruth Bridgewater* 28

A Story from a Sealed Room *Jeffrey M. Borkan* 30

The Knock on the Door at Night *Bob Stever* 32

Chapter 2. Suffering and Shame

Reflections *Howard F. Stein* 35

The Reluctant Samaritan *Kami Kandola* 40

Grace *Mindy Smith* 42

Newfound Lands *Ann C. Macaulay* 44

Beyond the Lock *Hans Antonneau* 46

Chapter 3. Learning from Patients

Reflections *Jack H. Medalie* 49

Melanie: The Path to Admiration *Frances Griffiths* 52

Passing: The "Norm" and Quality of Life *Mindy Smith* 54

Appearances   *William R. Phillips*   56

"Olga": A Quadriplegic and Living Alone   *Thomas M. Mettee*   57

The Alternative Cancer Patient   *Stanley G. Smith*   60

Restoring the Soul   *William L. Miller*   64

Chapter 4. Family and Community

Reflections   *Howard Brody*   67

Sleepless Nights   *Jack H. Medalie*   73

A Religious and Ethical Dilemma   *Robert C. Like*   78

Family Curse: "The Psychosomatic and the Danger of Death"
Dominique Huas   80

Last Day in Omak   *Jon O. Neher*   84

The Undertaker   *Igor Svab*   89

An IUD with a Special Meaning   *Aya Biderman*   91

Chapter 5. Humor

Reflections   *Justin Allen and Jeffrey M. Borkan*   95

Once upon a Time in the Land of Rock and Roll   *Peter Curtis*   98

Healers: The Physician and the Mori   *Michael Weingarten*   103

Magic and Technology   *Justin Allen*   104

She Laughed   *Perle Feldman*   107

William Tell and Me: A General Practitioner on Stage
Benedikt P. Horn   109

Chapter 6. Abuse

Reflections   *Carol P. Herbert and Shmuel Reis*   111

Revenge Is Sweet   *Judith Hollis-Triantafillou*   114

Music to Her Ears   *John C. Gunzburg*   117

What Doesn't Meet the Eye   *Hava Tabenkin*   121

Chapter 7. Suicide

Reflections   *Shimon Glick, Shmuel Reis, and Jeffrey M. Borkan*   125

Felo-de-se   *Robin Hull*   128

Going Round in the Wind   *Csaba Arnold*   131

Cyber-Family Practice: A Story in Three Parts   *Robert C. Like*   136

The Hand of Life   *Dov Steinmetz*   140

Chapter 8. Death

Reflections   *Kathy Cole-Kelly*   143

The Next Generation   *Stanley G. Smith*   147

The Farmer's Thumb   *Robin Hull*   150

Venancio's Legacy   *Mario Ahrens*   154

The Promise: A Love Story   *Perle Feldmun*   160

Jaw Pain and Panic: What to Do When Patients Consulting You Die in the Seat Belt   *Ivar Ostergaard*   163

Mr. Jones Needs to Be DNR'ed   *Kurt C. Stange*   165

Chapter 9. Secrets

Reflections   *Aya Biderman, Jeffrey M. Borkan, and Shmuel Reis*   169

The Hidden Patient: An Incident That Changed My Professional Life   *Jack H. Medalie*   172

A Hidden Fear   *Kurt C. Stange*   175

Tincture of Time   *Carol P. Herbert*   177

Unresolved Grief   *Walter W. Rosser*   179

Cancer, Lies, and Pathology Reports   *Mory Summer*   181

Chapter 10. Illness in the Doctor's Family

Reflections   *Jon O. Neher*   183

Uncommon Courage   *Howard F. Stein*   186

Confessions from the Heart   *Walter L. Larimore and Katherine Lee Larimore*   189

Birth, Death, and Music   *Mats Falk*   191

"You Be the Husband and Let Me Be the Doctor"   *Michael Klein*   195

Scars   *Michael Malus*   199

Epilogue   *Jeffrey M. Borkan and William L. Miller*   203
Contributors   209

Prologue

There are stories that patients tell. There are stories that doctors tell. Some doctors' stories are about patients; some about themselves. Some are written for a professional audience; some—so-called war stories—are meant for more intimate acquaintances. *Patients and Doctors* is composed of short tales from the clinic or from the home. They come to us from North America, from Europe, from Israel, from Africa. Some are about patients; some are about doctors; quite a few are about the encounters between patient and doctor.

These short stories vary in tone, in style, in meaning, and in quality of writing. Their purposes differ; so do their effects. The commentaries pull or push them in different directions. What we learn is less about the patient and family's experience of illness than it is about the experience of doctoring: how the doctor feels, thinks, practices. Thus we learn about patients from the perspective of the doctor. What is most arresting in these medical cameos is what they have to tell us about the ordinary and the extraordinary in the human affairs of treating sick people and being influenced by their lives.

We learn about the aesthetics of doctoring: things that happen in life that make the healer feel good or bad, and his or her practice feel graced with beauty or scarred with misadventure. We learn also about what is at stake in doctoring, including those things that morally matter and other things that in retrospect are laughable or absurd. Perhaps we learn most about how doctors formulate stories, tell them, and use them for professional or personal purposes. Stories become a part of therapeutic practices, mirroring their role in religion in devotional practices. Both are about creating transformation.

This collection leads me to wonder: what do doctors really want? Some of us seem to need divergence and diversity; others sameness, order, and stability. Some want danger; others serenity. We all seem to want (or demand) experiences that matter, but maybe what is foremost is that we want experiences in which *we* matter. Yet so many of the stories in this book conjure up the presence of others that maybe what we want above all is to show our usefulness and solidarity with others, to show, that is, *how* we matter. This—our suffering on behalf of those who suffer—is what Emmanuel Levinas, one of the great philosophers of the twentieth century, suggests creates the moral basis of human responses to suffering for us.

However, there are other "presences" in these stories, including a presence that comes close to a religious experience. We want, it seems, to document that meaning matters, that we are doing something whose importance lies in its intersubjective meaning, that that presence of shared meaning lends a sacred quality to the medical calling.

But what an odd lot we are! How different is the resonance of our words and the wording of what resonates for us. How strange is our privileged vision of life, when compared to the thousands of ways of being human. When we look hard at the world, how many others, outside of medicine and the professions broadly conceived, take for granted that healing is the primary task? That doing well is doing good by (and for) others? Perhaps our oddness is best shown in our sensibility of being wounded, incomplete, or failed, as much as successful, healers. In the therapeutic excesses of popular discourse in North America it is arresting and important to hear healers' uncertainty about therapeutic outcomes. We know, that is, that suffering is as certain in the human life course as tragedy is in the history of societies. Sometimes therapeutic transformation means transforming our therapeutic expectations to allow room for failure, for limitation, for endurance, for health.

Primary care is "primary" in several senses, not least because it gives access to firsthand experiences of suffering, witnessing, enduring, transcending. Stories are not just reflections of those existential experiences; they create them and change them too. We embed success in our therapeutic talk with patients, that is, we present a successful story line that we hope our patients can follow. We tell stories out of "court" (or clinic) to engage and remoralize others and ourselves.

Stories open up new paths, sometimes send us back to old ones, and close off still others. Telling (and listening to) stories we too imaginatively walk down those paths—paths of longing, paths of hope, paths of desperation. We are, actually, all of us, physicians and patients and family members too, storied folk: stories are what we are; telling and listening to stories is what we do. The stories in this collection evoke that existential quality.

ARTHUR KLEINMAN

Cambridge, Massachusetts

Acknowledgments

This book could not have been brought to light without the contributions, support, and love of countless individuals. Thanks must begin with the story writers and commentators. We received more than a hundred stories from physician writers around the world, who gave us hope that the human side of medicine is still very much "alive and well." Many individuals helped to guide this book's development and we are particularly indebted to Professors Sharon Kaufman and William Miller and to Ms. Rosalie Robertson and her assistants at the University of Wisconsin Press. Many others deserve our heartfelt thanks for the long hours spent editing and critiquing, from Irving Slott, Florence Yudkin, Jackie and Bill Schmidt, Lucille Falkoff, Madeleine and Ernest Jacobs, Carolyn and Norman Borkan, Terri Chebot, Suzanne Jacobs, Allison Hill, Debra Miller, Richard Juran, Miriam Erez and Keturah volunteers, Margaret Sills and Kelly Phillips.

The editors have their personal dedications, but we must start with those who gave us the sense of wonderment and awe for stories: our parents, teachers, colleagues, and patients. And to Professor Engel, from whom our inspiration springs.

Jeffrey Borkan: I dedicate this book to my family whose love has been the "story of my life," from my parents, siblings, and extended family; to my wife Suzanne who has supported me every step; to my continuing "narratives" and joys, my children, Ariela, Noa, and Aidan. The support, wisdom, and humanity of my community, from Kibbutz Deturah to Ben-Gurion University, to my patients in the Aravah, has been greatly cherished.

Shmuel Reis: To Noa, who is there for me continuously, in love. To Rachel, Yativ, Elyia, Roni, Zohar, and Gal, my loved and loving children. To my parents, Yaffa and the late Avraham, who taught me tederness and resilience. To Tomi and Chava, mentors and colleagues, and to many others—colleagues, students, and most of all patients—who shared stories of what life and healing is all about.

Jack Medalie: Thanks for the support of my wife, June, and to my patients who made my professional life interesting, stimulating, and very rewarding.

Dov Steinmetz: I dedicate the book to my sons: Oz, Alon, and Nir who are a constant source of inspiration and concern to me. To my parents, Ozer and Miriam, no longer among the living, yet always with me when I need them.

Patients and Doctors

Storytelling in Medicine

Jeffrey M. Borkan and William L. Miller

In the middle of a busy clinic morning, a fifty-six-year-old woman arrives for a consultation. The young family practitioner checks her chart and notes that she has diabetes and suffered a heart attack three years ago, followed by a triple coronary artery bypass. She has been to the clinic frequently in the last few months, but the physician has found little to explain her symptoms. Short and overweight, she is dressed in a simple, well-worn dress and kerchief, and possesses the worried, sculpted facial lines of one who has known hard work and hardship.

She has lived alone since her husband died and her children married and moved to their own houses. She feels heaviness in her chest and upper abdomen, which she describes as pulsing, throbbing, and gnawing. The symptoms are worse after the sun goes down, and sometimes she feels very anxious. She is concerned that these attacks will kill her, and she mumbles something about "peace in heaven." The doctor politely listens, checks her blood pressure, pulse, heart, and lungs, and orders an electrocardiogram (EKG). When he returns to the room after a few minutes, he reviews the EKG and reassures the patient that it is normal and that the pains are probably "musculoskeletal body aches."

He gives her a prescription for an anti-inflammatory drug, but as he begins to rise to leave the room, the patient reaches for his arm and quietly implores, "I have to tell you something else. . . ." With an inaudible sigh and a look at his watch, the doctor sits back down. The woman then recounts the story of her fourth pregnancy, twenty years earlier, when she gave birth to a stillborn fetus near term. Although the death of this child was due to natural causes, she considered herself responsible. Times had been hard, the pregnancy was unplanned, and she had been ambivalent about having another baby when her first children were already teenagers.

At the time, her heart was "empty of love" for this unborn child; however, since the stillbirth, she has suffered from a sense of guilt, which had grown over the years. Since the heart attack, she has heard voices and feels that the spirit of the child has been tormenting her, repaying her for her "sin." She believes that she must join the child in heaven, where she might be able to mother it and provide the love she had denied it before.

Storytelling

The telling of stories is a basic element of human life, an integral part of daily existence. Throughout our waking hours, we hear and recount endless narratives. We relate our dreams, read the morning paper, provide instructive anecdotes to co-workers, entrust secret confidences, listen to our children's school tales, watch television dramas, and describe the day's events. For both the teller and the listener, there is a natural compulsion to share information. Storytelling gives shape to current experience, recounts and gives meaning to the past, and attempts to foretell and reduce anxiety regarding the future.

Storytelling in Medicine

In medicine, storytelling has a long history. Clinical accounts of individual cases were once the primary medium of medical knowledge (Hunter 1991). The great classical physicians from Hippocrates to Osler conveyed their "pearls" as prose in compelling stories of illness. A look at their writings and at the accounts of their teaching gives an indication of the elegance of their narrative skills. Medical journals of 1798 had greater literary flavor, readability, and power to engage the reader than their dry, if more scientific, offspring today.

The Decline of Storytelling

Somewhere along the way, physicians have lost or at least neglected their ability to listen to and tell stories. So many patients complain, "Doctor, you're not listening to me," and they are often right. After inundating patients with the accumulated knowledge of particular diagnoses, often in "medicalese," medical students, residents, and senior clinicians cannot understand why patients leave appearing more confused and depressed than before. As in the preceding vignette, medical personnel all too commonly extract the signs and symptoms of "chest pain" from the rich and varied context of life's drama, ignoring the person and the individual suffering. The patient may be seen as the sum of his or her pathophysiology until part of the story jars our steady biomedical gaze and forces us to refocus on the whole person—if we pay attention.

Although privileged to hear the intimate stories of others' lives, many physicians allow little time for expression and convert patients' narratives into symptom checklists. Research has documented that physicians give patients an average of eighteen seconds to tell their stories before interrupting and diverting the focus on to doctor-oriented disease topics (Beckman and Frankel 1984). Even those introductions that seemed interminably long to the physician seldom exceeded two minutes.

This neglect has a number of causes. Clinical teaching using individual cases, prominent until this century, has been replaced by scientific theory and classifications of symptoms and disease. The growth of "technomedicine" since World War II has paralleled, and perhaps prompted, the decline of the humanistic side of healing, of which stories are a part. Although they did not

4

disappear, stories were labeled with two of the most pejorative terms in medicine, "anecdotal" and "unscientific." In her book *Doctors' Stories,* Hunter points out that this may be appropriate: "The number and variety of signs and symptoms observed and reported by the ill render the single case a deceptive guide to understanding disease in another human being, even the same disease in a second patient" (1991:70). Since stories in medicine are concerned only with the single instance, their fallibility and power to deceive are high. Acting on the basis of personal experience or the individual case contravenes the epidemiological basis of modern medicine, particularly the current version of "evidence-based clinical practice." Anecdotes and stories, personalized and particularistic, may well lead to errors in diagnosis and treatment if generalized. The evidence-based physician is instructed to act on the basis of depersonalized "hard data," such as those derived from randomized clinical trials. In addition, listening to stories may be seen as "inefficient," taking away from more "essential" patient care activities, especially in the "time-driven" managed care era.

The Centrality of Narrative in Clinical Encounters

Medical stories did not and could not disappear, however, since they are a fundamental part of health care. Unlike other scientific and humanistic disciplines, clinical medicine is dependent on narrative. Stories and storytelling are central to the clinical encounter where both the patient and the physician process their personal experiences by putting them into words (Borkan, Miller, and Reis 1992; Greenhalgh and Hurwitz 1999).

The clinical encounter can be conceptualized as cooperative doctor–patient storytelling with openings, complications, and resolutions. Stories exist within a particular sociomedical context, itself governed by rules and etiquette. Patients and clinicians enter consultations with expectations of how the conversation will proceed. Each expects the other to conform to his or her "rules" and becomes impatient, dissatisfied, and angry if these are broken (Herman 1990; Borkan, Miller, and Reis 1992). Patients open with their chief concerns, histories, and illness problems, conveyed in limitless range and style. These narratives reflect how they have pieced together and made sense of events within and around them, guided by their own past experiences and those of others.

Although the variation and multiplicity of patient stories make clinical practice a continuing source of excitement, such accounts may be unwieldy and patients are encouraged by their physicians and by the outpatient milieu to present a condensed, chronological version of their distress and suffering. Physicians enter the story with additional twists, complications, and insights. They often counter their patients' chronicles with a professionally molded, finite set of diagnostic categories, the official medical "plot lines." As an overlay on patients' unique stories, most physicians, regardless of specialty, use only a few score of diagnoses, defined by previous professional socialization and developments in the medical literature. Physicians reformulate the story according to their professionalized model of medical care, occasionally sharing this version with the patient.

Further reformulations may occur as patient and physician negotiate treatments and diagnostic plans. Plot lines must be interwoven and the dissimilarities between patient and physician stories must be adjusted so that there is general agreement on the resolution stage of the medical narrative—usually the need for further diagnostic tests and/or treatments. The implicit or explicit negotiations to reach closure may mean patients leave the physician's office with an antibiotic for an upper respiratory infection even though that was not part of the doctor's original story ending or that the patient reframes his or her misery on to a more hopeful story line. Finally, after resolution is achieved, the story is presented again. The two parties record the details the interaction and its meaning—the patient in his or her memory and the physician in the charts.

The Persistence of Medical Narratives in Clinical Thought and Teaching

In addition to their role in the medical encounter, clinical narrative or anecdotes allow clinicians to bridge the epistemological divide between the general rules of disease, the "classic cases" described in textbooks, and the particular factors of an individual patient's illness (Hunter 1991). As Hunter reminds us, "Medicine is filled with stories. The imperfect fit between biological knowledge and the expression and treatment of disease in the individual leaves room for variants, surprises, anomalies. These are events, noteworthy occurrences. . . . Unexpected clinical phenomena" (pp. 69–70). Narratives have also been given greater attention by adherents to the "biopsychosocial model," "family-systems," and "holistic" medical approaches (Engel 1977; Glenn 1988; White 1988; Antonovsky 1989; Herman 1990). These approaches see the narrative as an expression of medicine that extends beyond the molecular, cellular, and organ levels to include the person, the family, and the society, which, as Engel points out, can and should also be considered "scientific" (Engel 1977).

Medical narratives have remained the currency of informal physician communication, from private anecdotes whispered in hospital hallways to the bits of the day shared with family members at home. An evening spent in a social gathering of doctors is filled with their storytelling, often about the personalities and problems of their patients. We tell and retell stories at every stage of training, throughout our professional lives. In addition to the cases formally presented to students, residents, and professors during the clinical portion of a physician's education, informal stories of solved or unsolved difficult cases are the stuff of professional and quasi-social discourse (Hunter 1991).

Stories cannot be eliminated from teaching, either. Though many contemporary lecturers attempt to convey knowledge and understanding through citing overarching principles and theories, the most effective teachers use illustrative cases to provide an informative and entertaining bridge to general scientific knowledge (Hunter 1986; Brody 1987). Stories spark and hold our interest in a way dry exposition of theory never can achieve. Even when presented in a flattened monotone, they nonetheless assign a human face to disease mechanisms. Though often not considered noteworthy in and of themselves, the more unusual of these anecdotes provide the raw material for morbidity and mortality rounds, case presentations, and problem-oriented teaching. Clinician-teachers who tell stories—especially if they are from their own clinical encounters—can stimulate students to examine their attitudes and values in a way that may be impossible to achieve by other methods (Hensel and Rasco 1992).

The Rebirth of Medical Story Writing

Fortunately, medical storytelling has undergone a rebirth in the professional and lay literature. Physicians with an impulse to write frequently condense their experiences and their medical careers into collections of stories, endlessly drawn upon to provide authoritative examples. The popularity of books by Oliver Sacks, Robert Coles, John Stone, John McPhee, Sharon Kaufman, and Michael Malus reflects a zest for stories by physicians. Among physicians, there has been a growth of and demand for story columns in medical journals (Charon 1994).

Physician Stories as Representations

All of the narratives in this book are "physician stories," written in the medical voice. This medical voice (or "voice of medicine") represents "the technical-scientific assumptions of medicine," as distinguished from the "voice of the life-world, which is the natural attitude of everyday life" (Mishler 1984:14). The stories emerge from the vivid memories of family physicians educated in Western biomedicine. These stories reflect more than just physicians' recollections of memorable encounters. They reflect what physicians are willing to tell about themselves, reveal about themselves. Narratives should not to be confused with real events, facts, or recordings of what occurred in the flow of clinical practice and everyday life (Young 1982; Kaufman 1997). Rather, they are *reconstructions* and *representations* of events which the storyteller fashions in a presentational manner, deliberate descriptions which engage the listener. Stories account for ways in which physician-narrators remember, describe, and engage an event or problem (Kaufman 1997). The *truths* in narratives, as in ethnographic writing, are inherently *partial*, constrained by the incompleteness of the representational process

(Clifford 1986). One can never "tell it all," nor does any version have sole claim to "reality" or "truth."

Medical stories do not emanate from a vacuum. The stories and their narrators are influenced by a host of factors which govern their structure, language, cadence, and insights, not the least of which is medical professionalization and socialization (Good 1995). Like ethnographic writing (Clifford 1986), what we finally see in the physician-writer's narrative is determined in at least seven ways:

1. Contextually: the story draws from a social milieu.
2. Rhetorically: the narrative uses accepted conventions for written expression.
3. Institutionally: physician-storytellers write from within (and/or against) specific traditions, schools of thought, disciplines, audiences.
4. Generically: different types of writing have different distinguishable styles, that is, stories are different from travelogues or journal reports.
5. Politically: the authority with which one writes and represents events is unequally shared, with frequently contested issues, such as "whose version" will be accepted.
6. Developmentally: the physician-storyteller changes in terms of his or her personal, professional, and literary development over time.
7. Historically: all of the above are constantly changing, in a fluid and dynamic process.

Content of This Book

This book represents an effort to further the narrative trend in medicine and thereby stimulate the sharing of the intimate mysteries of our work. It constitutes an international effort to explore the value of narratives in primary care through the compilation of family and general practice physicians' most memorable stories. Some of the contributors are internationally recognized professors and physician-writers. Some are country or urban doctors known only to their patients. What they have in common is sensitivity to the story and an ability to convey it through their words. Though this collection is designed principally for primary health care providers, its goal is to be sufficiently accessible to attract the lay reader and sufficiently engaging to interest behavioral scientists, anthropologists, and sociologists.

Each storyteller offers insights into the conflicts, challenges, and exaltations of primary care. Some stories provide transcendence, touching on themes which are larger than the writer or the subject—life, death, joy, sadness, community. Some stories mark breakthroughs in the personal and professional development of the doctor—critical junctures that change the provider forever. In general, the stories are from experienced family doctors, committed to the biopsychosocial model of care. This concept originated with Engel (1977), who, believing that traditional biomedicine was in crisis due to its adherence to "a model of disease no longer adequate for scientific tasks and social responsibilities," proposed a new biopsychosocial medical model. This new model pays explicit attention to "humanness" (Engel 1996) and describes a person as an integrated mix of biological, psychological, and social dimensions. The biopsychosocial model considers the individual with the disease, as well as the disease itself, for example, "the unique personal features of the patient, the doctor–patient relationship, the family, the community, and the spiritual dimension" (Smith 1996). In this paradigm, the mind and body are not separable, requiring the health professional to deal with the whole person. Though there are great differences between the stories, particularly in regard to their sense of humility, awe, and comfort with complexity, uncertainty, and ambiguity, they are widely committed to the biopsychosocial model of care and have a "good ear" for the narrative.

Stories are grouped by themes into chapters, each beginning with a reflection. By this exercise, we hope to harness the universal power of stories within a didactic framework. We also hope to portray the voice of primary care physicians—something rarely done in a specialist-dominated world. These themes contribute to the growing literature of medical narratives that may enhance the humanness of the practitioner and may provide material for teaching students and residents. They may strengthen the resolve of weary physicians to go on; they may inspire some to put their own stories on paper. They may also hearten patients by introducing physicians who think, feel, and care.

The Local and the Universal

Why compile stories from around the world? We see the book as a kind of journey, both for the story writers and for the readers. For the writer, putting the story into words is often a pilgrim's path to expression and understanding of experience. The reader is whisked from the jungles of Cambodia to the icy tundra of Canada's Northwest Territories to the squalor of urban American poverty. However, the particular social, cultural, physical, and temporal settings are merely the background, the "experience-near," for the interplay of events and the vivid portrayal of larger human conflicts and exaltations.

By examining the individual struggles of physicians with patients, illnesses, and their own strengths and limitations, we are privileged to catch a glimpse of local worlds, knowledge, and experience. The writers in this book have generally been very successful in providing a sense of locality. As Appadurai, an anthropologist, has recently noted, "The production of locality . . . is not simply a matter of producing local subjects as well as the very neighborhoods that contextualize their subjectivities . . . [in addition] space and time are themselves socialized and localized through complex and deliberate practices of performance, representation, and action" (1996:180).

This book presents dramatic stories about doctor–patient relationships, often within the context of marked social and cultural differences. When we refer to *culture,* we are not simply delineating objects, things, or substances, whether physical or metaphysical (Appadurai 1996). This older definition becomes entangled with notions of race, biological kinship, genealogy, and territoriality. Rather we are adopting a more contemporary redefinition of culture that does not simply stress the possession of certain attributes, whether material, linguistic, or geographic. Instead it focuses on the "consciousness of these attributes and their naturalization as essential to group identity," with the core of the concept of ethnicity resting on "the conscious and imaginative construction and mobilization of *differences* as its core" (Appadurai 1996:13–14).

Although the representation of local worlds, knowledge, and experience is a valuable achievement in itself, the stories do not stop there but also succeed in connecting with transcendent universal themes. The experience of physicians in their local worlds strikes cords of identification with health care providers' struggles everywhere. The problems the physician-writers face and their responses to these situations provide a glimpse both at the milieu in which they function and at the unique elements which the stories portray: sadness, joy, struggles against adversity, sense of satisfaction at one's chosen avocation.

Types of Stories

Arthur Frank, in *The Wounded Storyteller* (1995), suggests that Western physicians seek, almost need, what he calls *restitution narratives.* Physicians desperately want their stories to have clear resolutions, which ideally involve full restoration of patients to original health. Many of these stories reveal the bias of this framework of understanding. There is a strong desire for the storytellers to find restitution, and discomfort occurs when there is none or threatens to be none. Most of the physician-writers who contributed to this book, and the vast majority who appear in the professional and lay press, neatly wrap up their stories into discrete packages with clear openings, defined complications, and tidy endings. This is particularly true in the "hero narratives" of Chapter 1, in which the physician intervenes between life and death.

There are other stories in which structurally the narrative has no closure or the end to the story is neither satisfying nor clear. For example, a few of the contributions in this book, such as those by Drs. Biderman, Tabenkin, Stanley Smith, and Malus, stand alone as such "quest narratives," where the writer is still on the path and the final outcome is not yet in sight. "Failure narratives," where the physicians portray their inability to heal or to form a therapeutic alliance, are less frequently shared, both in professional life and in this book. One such story, a touching saga of the death of a young patient, was offered by a seasoned family physician and teacher, only to be withdrawn from publication as the doctor contemplated how peers and the local community might view the tragedy. Dr. Medalie bravely offers a similar perspective in the second of his contributions. In this story, he reports how he tells the truth to his patient, only to be left alone feeling helpless and confused, the therapeutic relationship unraveled, with no clear path to restore it. But was there no healing? The family and friends of the barren woman left wailing, tearing their clothes, and throwing sand upon themselves. Could this represent a step on the quest for healing an unavoidable tragedy? How do we wail, tear our clothes, and throw sand upon ourselves? Many hold their failures inside, allowing them to smolder and decay; others step into self-destructive habits; others tell stories.

How to Approach These Stories

Initially it is the comparison between settings and societies that demands our attention. Then it is the writer and his or her hidden assumptions suddenly revealed which hold these stories irrevocably in the memories of their tellers—and, we hope, yours. These stories may be a looking glass through which we see ourselves and our moral dilemmas more clearly.

The stories in this book may awaken our own questions: What knowledge and mystery are present in our patients and in our encounters and are we able to learn from them? What do we glean from the context of care? What types of patient–physician relationships and alliances do we form, what influences them, and are they beneficial for healing? What are the challenges of our profession and are we able to meet them? How do we deal with the unexpected? With failure? How do we cope with the pressures of caring for others or the pressures of illness in our own families? Are we open to the *other*, whether in terms of person, experience, or milieu? Do we create sufficient space for the *other* in our clinical encounters and healing relationships? Are we open to ourselves? Have our own growth and development been enhanced through our work or are we stuck?

The goal of this book is the enjoyment, growth, and stimulation of the reader. We hope that the reader, upon encountering the stories of family and general physicians struggling with their own strengths and limitations, will benefit from the richness of description of the local worlds and gain fuller understanding of healing, the healers, and, ultimately, of themselves. These are also courageous tales. They come from authors who have the moral courage to risk exposing the dilemmas they faced. We hope that this book will touch your heart and head: surprising you, engaging you emotionally, and stimulating you intellectually. Regardless of whether you are comforted or disturbed by what you read, we hope that the stories will challenge you morally and intellectually, leaving you more aware, and less certain.

References

Antonovsky, A. 1989. Islands rather than bridgeheads: the problematic status of the biopsychosocial model. *Family Systems Medicine* 7(3):243–53.

Appadurai, A. 1996. *Modernity at Large: Cultural Dimensions of Globalization.* Minneapolis: University of Minnesota Press.

Beckman, H. B., and R. M. Frankel. 1984. The effect of physician behavior on the collection of data. *Annals of Internal Medicine* 101:692–96.

Borkan, J. M., W. L. Miller, and S. Reis. 1992. Medicine as storytelling. *Family Practice* 9:127–29.

Brody, H. 1987. *Stories of Sickness.* New Haven: Yale University Press.

Charon, R. 1994. The internist reading: doctors at the heart of the novel. *Annals of Internal Medicine* 121(5):390–91.

Clifford, J. 1986. Introduction: Partial Truths. In J. Clifford and G. Marcus (eds.). *Writing Culture: The Poetics and Politics of Ethnography.* Berkeley: University of California Press, pp. 1–26.

Coles, R. 1989. *The Call of Stories: Teaching and the Moral Imagination.* Boston: Houghton Mifflin.

Engel, G. L. 1977. The need for a new medical model: a challenge for biomedicine. *Science* 196:129–36.

Engel, G. L. 1996. From biomedical to biopsychosocial: 1. Being scientific in the human domain. *Family Systems and Health* 14:425–33.

Frank, A. W. 1995. *The Wounded Storyteller: Body, Illness, and Ethics.* Chicago: University of Chicago Press.

Glenn, M. 1988. The resurgence of the biomedical model in medicine. *Family Systems Medicine* 6(4):492–500.

Good, M. J. D. 1995. *American Medicine: The Quest for Competence.* Berkeley: University of California Press.

Greenhalgh, T., and D. Hurwitz. 1999. Why study narrative. *British Medical Journal* 318:48–50.

Hensel, W. A., and T. L. Rasco. 1992. Storytelling as a method for teaching values and attitudes. *Academic Medicine* 67:500–4.

Herman, J. 1990. Anger in the consultation. *British Journal of General Practice,* May, pp. 176–77.

Hunter, K. 1986. "There was this one guy . . .": the uses of anecdotes in medicine. *Perspectives in Biology and Medicine* 29:619–30.

Hunter, K. M. 1991. *Doctors' Stories: The Narrative Structure of Medical Knowledge.* Princeton, NJ: Princeton University Press.

Kaufman, S. R. 1988. Stroke Rehabilitation and the Negotiation of Identity. In S. Reinharz and G. D. Rowles (eds.). *Qualitative Gerontology.* New York: Springer, pp. 82–103.

Kaufman, S. R. 1993. *The Healer's Tale.* Madison: University of Wisconsin Press.

Kaufman, S. R. 1997. Construction and practice of medical responsibility: dilemmas and narratives from geriatrics. *Culture, Medicine and Psychiatry* 21(1):1–26.

Kleinman, A. 1980. *Patients and Healers in the Context of Culture.* Berkeley: University of California Press.

Lehrman, N. S. 1993. Pleasure heals: the role of social pleasure—love in its broadest sense—in medical practice. *Archives of Internal Medicine* 153:929–34.

Malus, M. 1994. *Before the End of the Day: Stories from a Doctor's Journal.* Montreal, Quebec: Vehicule Press.

McPhee, J. 1984. *Heirs of General Practice.* New York: Farrar, Straus and Giroux.

Mishler, E. G. 1984. *The Discourse of Medicine: Dialetics of Medical Interviews.* Norwood, NJ: Ablex.

Smith, R. C. 1996. *The Patient's Story.* Boston: Little Brown.

White, K. L. 1988. *The Task of Medicine: Dialogue at Wickenburg.* Menlo Park, Calif.: Henry J. Kaiser Family Foundation.

Young, K. 1982. Edgework: frame and boundary in the phenomenology of narrative communication. *Semiotica* 41:277–315.

Young, K. 1997. *Presence in the Flesh: The Body in Medicine.* Cambridge, Mass.: Harvard University Press.

Beyond the Call of Duty

Reflections

Robin Hull

The dominant theme in this chapter's stories may best be introduced by telling an experience of visiting a grave a few miles from my home in the beautiful Scottish county of Perthshire, part of the ancient township of Weem. The village there is dominated by one of the finest sixteenth-century castles in Scotland, the home and center of Clan Menzies. Not far from the castle the auld kirk, built in 1600, serves as a mausoleum for past members of this great family. In the kirk there are many memorials to the dead members of the clan. I have to confess that when I first read the epitaph on the stone of Anne, Lady Menzies (1822–1878), wife of Sir Robert Menzies, Seventh Baronet, I laughed aloud. The inscription read "She hath done what she could." At first sight this seems to be the epitome of damnation by faint praise. Further thought, however, led me to realize what the obituarist had meant.

Nineteenth-century life in Highland Scotland was often nasty, brutish, and short. Poverty, apart from clan chiefs, was universal, and people lived in simple, dark, damp, smoky hovels where disease was rife, killing many children before their tenth birthdays. Hunger was not unusual, and great famines, as occurred in Ireland, were mirrored in Scotland (Keay and Keay 1994). The clan organization was paramount in this existence. Paternalistic chiefs cared for their people, some better than others, and in turn the men of the clan served them even unto death as tenants, servants, and fighting soldiers. Among clan leaders some chiefs, and their ladies, were devoted to their people and did all they could to improve the lot of the common man. So "to hath done what she could" in the face of such a harsh environment was far from faint praise. Had the mason cut "would" or "should" instead of "could" on her tombstone, an entirely different message would have been left. "Would" suggests at best arrogant selfishness, at worst libertinism. "Should" implies an inhuman adherence to duty in the face of indifference to the suffering of the people. The use of "could" tells us that she cared and did her best for them in the face of great difficulty. Lady Anne did what she could because her personality and upbringing demanded that she should.

The editors grouped five stories under the heading "Beyond the Call of

Duty" and even suggested that I should look at references connected with heroism in medicine. I suppose the phrase "beyond the call of duty" is redolent of Victoria Crosses and Purple Hearts, and yet the essays they sent me were not like that at all. These are tales concerning normal clinical experiences, albeit under highly abnormal circumstances, and I felt certain that none of their authors would claim the appellation "hero" as a result of their accounts.

But the stories do have a theme—one which is extremely relevant to primary care both in its past and, even more particularly, in its future. Our branch of medicine is intensely pragmatic; as physicians we have to do *what is possible,* often under the far from ideal circumstances of the patient's own environment. That is exactly what the storytellers in this chapter did. A house call to transfer a child with appendicitis to a hospital, cardiopulmonary resuscitation, care of the first stage of labor, even the treatment of pneumonia in an infant are all part of the task of primary care. But look at the setting of these tales— the local context.

Perhaps most readers will not appreciate the full severity of the situation Dr. Ratulangie describes. To understand its significance one has to know that in Holland—particularly Zeeland, where most of the land is below sea level— the outflow of the great rivers that drain northwest Europe has to be carefully controlled by a system of dikes and pumping stations. The area is astonishing for the incredible sophistication of the Rijkswaterstaat defenses which the Netherlands built after the floods of January 1953 when more than a thousand died in a single night. On such a night of catastrophe struggling through the circumstances to arrange a much-needed appendectomy was indeed "doing what one could."

When Saddam Hussein sent twenty-six scud missiles into Israel in January 1991 he was attempting to precipitate the entry of Israel into war in the hope that the Islamic nations would then support his attempt to destroy the Jewish state. At the time it was believed that these missiles were armed with chemical, bacteriological, and possibly nuclear warheads. So, as we join Dr. Borkan in his sealed room with his family and a woman in labor while full-scale Middle-eastern war hung in balance, we may share his conflict of emotion and duty to his patient. To those of us remote from the Gulf War (though hardly stirring as our television screens presented the local situation and experience to a global audience), the Iraqi bombardment of Israel did not seem too bad—we heard that most missiles were destroyed before reaching their targets and that those that did arrive caused little harm. Yet we know the media distort reality and experience, often making light of dangerous circumstances while inflating the dangers of minor incidents. However, to be at the receiving end of unknown quantities and qualities of mass destruction must be terrifying indeed.

Retreating with the Borkan family into their shelter, quelling the fear of the children, and wondering about gas, biological, or radiation threat one can appreciate the horror of the night described. As if paternal duties were not

16

enough, there was the patient in labor. Interestingly, amid all the fear and drama, there was time to reflect on the experience of a delivery on the children, who, in that confined space, must be the most intimate spectators. Perhaps the physician was the most fortunate person in that sealed room; we must all have experienced times when the anxiety of clinical situations has relieved, or at least blotted out, pressing worries in our own personal lives.

The body's struggle for survival and physicians' reaction to it is well described in the two tales of cardiopulmonary resuscitation. This is a commonplace event in hospitals, but many heart attacks occur in public places where the doctor is present by chance and armed with nothing but the hands and the skill with which to save life. Dr. Reis experienced this at Ben-Gurion Airport. Unrecognized among the spectators at Ben-Gurion Airport was the patient's wife, witnessing the horror of attempted resuscitation and facing the imminent prospect of widowhood. It is hard at such times to spare essential seconds away from the patient to comfort the relatives. Yet it was from the moment that the doctors managed to comfort the wife that the patient's heart responded. The doctors did what they could and in so doing perhaps helped the wife to do what she could. Cold science may reject the power of prayer and love calling out to a failing myocardium, but at least two of the people at Ben-Gurion that day would disagree with such objectivity.

One can share the relief that Dr. Bridgewater felt when the "knights in the flashing white charger" took from her all responsibility after she had done what she could, and one can also feel the sting of irritation at the superiority of the uninvolved hospital doctor who suggested disparagingly that no arrest had occurred.

Dr. Stever has a different tale but one also set against war, this time in Southeast Asia. Here it was not just the doctor who did what he could, for a baby was saved through the devotion of his parents. It is remarkable that the poison arrow–toting Khmai Loer parents, with neither language nor medical experience in common with the physician, quickly learned to hold their dying infant and gave artificial respiration while the physician struggled with the difficult task of getting fluids into veins collapsed by dehydration. All did what they could, the child survived, and the reward for the sophistication of Western medicine was the ultimate of superstitious Cambodian good fortune, a tiger's claw. Clinical skill saved the child but one wonders what those parents felt about the part played by their faith in their tiger charm: did they believe it determined their arrival at Dr. Stever's hospital at the moment of crisis?

All these stories bring together one aspect of family doctoring: its intense pragmatism. This might be defined as the ability to find something that could be done in the face of need and seeming lack of resource. But the stories also illustrate the incredible bond that forms between the family doctor and his or her patient in times of crisis. Perhaps this bond is all the stronger when the doctor, rather than working as a technological miracle worker with drugs and procedures, makes due under unusual circumstances. Did the generally happy outcomes seen in these narratives result from fortune favoring these "accoucheurs," or was there some other factor based on such unscientific qualities of relationship as love, trust, and faith?

The stories also raise the question of motivation: *why* did the doctors do what they could? Like Lady Anne Menzies, their unconscious motivation lay in the complex blend of their personalities and their upbringing, in this case their professional training.

As medicine enters a new millennium doctors need to rethink the relationships that exist between them and their patients. Perhaps one of the most thought-provoking books published on this relationship in recent years is Edward Shorter's *Bedside Manners* (1985). Shorter carefully traces the history of the doctor–patient relationship from the days of the horse-and-buggy doctor to our own era. He draws on that wonderful painting by Sir Luke Fildes, *The Doctor* (1891), which hangs in the Tate Gallery in London, to illustrate the powerlessness of doctors against disease a century ago. This picture, so often used in medical teaching, has a fascinating history. The artist lost his own child to tuberculosis and wished to document some of the devotion of a doctor who did his best for the child in the face of this terrible infection. Fildes reconstructed in his London studio a Cornish fisherman's cottage, which he used for the background of the painting. He then recruited a number of London general practitioners to sit in relays for him until he found the exact quality that he wanted for his picture. Robin Downie, professor of medical ethics at Glasgow Medical School, in his anthology *The Healing Arts* (1993), comments on the result: "The painting is an elegant portrayal of what medicine is all about—the doctor, the patient, and the quality of the relationship that exists between them. The physician is attending the patient, watching and waiting—*being there* [emphasis added]. Much of the painting's impact is in the space between the physician's eyes and the child, which is filled, solely, by the doctor's gaze." One might add to this that current medical technology was represented in the picture by a bowl with a teaspoon in it.

Shorter uses this picture to illustrate the strength of quality of the doctor–patient bond that existed at a time when the doctor was really quite impotent against disease. He contrasts this with the strained relationships that exist a century later. That things have changed there can be no doubt. In the 1960s grateful patients in rural Britain plied their doctors with presents of food, wine, and other gifts; these gradually lessened through the seventies and eighties to become quite a rarity in the last decade of the century. Tangible expressions of the warmth of the relationship waned steadily. More seriously, although the interventions available today are immensely powerful, today's doctor is often abused, sometimes assaulted, and increasingly taken to court by dissatisfied patients. Clearly if primary care is to continue in the twenty-first century as the undoubtedly important branch of medicine that it is, this deterioration in relationships needs to be addressed.

Lady Anne Menzies's strange epitaph suggests how an understanding of the verbs *should* and *could* serve a useful way of examining this change in the doctor–patient relationship. In an age when doctors are seen by the laity as having a pill for every ill and thought of as having a duty to cure everything from infertility to senility, the gap between reality and expectation must grow ever wider. Of course the doctor *should* do whatever is reasonable to minimize human suffering, but if by doing so, and consuming vast resources, he limits what he *could* have done, where lies the sense?

This chapter's storytellers, like Lady Anne, did what they could because their personalities and training demanded of them that they should do so unquestioningly. This has lessons for all who are involved in medical education: we need to select and teach future doctors in a better way than we have so far accomplished. To live up to the meaning of the word *doctor,* the family physicians of the future must have the unquestioning desire to do what they can and the right training to give them the knowledge, skills, and attitudes to have much that they could do. For too long medical education has been so overfactual that essential qualities of communication, empathy, and an appreciation of the importance of "being there" have been discarded as so much "soft soap." Kerr White, when reporting "The Dialogue at Wickenburg," discussed the need to broaden the paradigm of medical education from one based on biochemical processes to include behavioral, environmental, and psychological aspects of disease (White 1988). In defining "a new kind of doctor" Tudor Hart looks to one who, though still scientific, has broadened the concept of medicine from Oslerian criteria to include a more dependable alliance with the patient (Hart 1988). It is encouraging to see that increasingly medical school curricula are coming to stress communication skills, ethics, and palliative care as never before, though not yet enough. Sir Luke Fildes's doctor was not so impotent after all—we need to emulate him just as our storytellers did.

Commentator's Note:
The letter from the editor of *Patients and Doctors* asking me to write a commentary on a clutch of these tales arrived just after I had an accident hill walking and had fractured my spine. Once initial pain was controlled, the chief inconvenience was immobility and I was maddened by frustration and inactivity. At first the editor's detailed instructions seemed an imposition, all the more so since he requested references to current literature relating to the theme of the stories. Initial irritation gave way before the realization that the task set me was, if nothing else, a useful therapy. Thus like Lady Menzies, I did what I could.

A Stormy Case of Appendicitis

C. J. Albert Ratulangie
Zevenbergen, The Netherlands

On Saturday night, January 31, 1953, I listened to a concert on the radio and went to bed as the wind howled around the house in Zevenbergen, a small town in the southern Netherlands. A few weeks earlier I had left the training hospital and had come to Zevenbergen to substitute in the practice of a colleague who had suffered a bleeding ulcer and was recovering at his parent's home in another part of the country. The nearest hospital was in Breda, about fifteen kilometers away. There were two general practitioners in Zevenbergen, taking weekend duties in rotation, and this was my weekend.

I was aroused by the urgent ringing of the doorbell. I switched on the light; my watch showed it was three o'clock in the morning. The howling of the wind had taken on a higher pitch. At the front door stood two men, presumably farmers. The elder one, apparently the father, said, "Sorry to trouble you this time of night, Doctor, but would you please come with us to have a look at my daughter? She is in terrible pain." I asked a few questions and found that the pain, which was in her lower belly, had started all of a sudden, and she had vomited once. I said, "All right, I will put some clothes on, get the car out of the garage, and follow you." "Oh, no, Doctor," the younger one said, "You can't get through in your car—the dike has broken and the roads are flooded. You'd better come with us in the jeep, and you'd better dress as warmly as you can."

I showed them into the waiting room and went upstairs to get dressed. Over my pajamas I put on a pair of slacks, a flannel shirt, a thick woolen sweater, and a windbreaker. After getting my black bag from the office, I went back to the waiting room. They looked me over, then the elder man said, "You will catch a bad cold in that, Doctor—do you realize there is a real gale blowing? Jaap will get something better." The younger man had already gone out and came back with a sort of ulster, really heavy and at least one size too big for me, but when we got out in the shrieking wind I was grateful.

The name Zevenbergen, literally translated, means "seven hills," and the town indeed is situated on a low hill, surrounded by polders (land reclaimed in the past centuries from the tidal delta, formed by the estuaries of the river Meuse, by the construction of dikes). We left the town and were driving over a dike. To the left and right, as far as one could see in the darkness, there was only windswept water. From time to time a wave would break against the dike and the wind would blow the spray against the windshield and into our faces. I hoped the dike would withstand the fury of the waves. Here and there one could see farmhouse lights reflected on the waves, like little islands in a vast expanse of water—an eerie sight.

The men told me that they were aroused at midnight by the dikewatch, which is always called to duty on nights like this, and told that the dike had broken and the water was rising fast. Then the family, along with the two farmhands, started to take their belongings to safety. They drove the bigger cattle, the cows and calves, to the dike and took the hens, pigs, and the lighter farming tools to the loft of the shed. Inside the house they were carrying as much as possible to the loft, when suddenly the farmer's daughter, Maria, uttered a cry of pain and immediately vomited. She doubled over in agony and all they could do was put her to bed, hoping it would wear off after a while. They had tried to get me on the phone, but the line was dead.

Eventually Jaap, the farmer's son, brought the jeep to a stop. In the water I could see, bobbing up and down in the waves, a rowboat tied to a tree. "We use that boat to go fishing on Sundays," explained the father. From under the front seat Jaap produced a pair of Wellington boots. "You'd better put those on, Doctor," he said. I did. They were a few sizes too large but I soon realized they would keep my feet dry anyway.

We got in the boat. I sat on the bottom at the bow, Jaap rowed, and the father held the tiller. It was a fairly comfortable trip, as we were going downwind. Occasionally I looked over my shoulder and saw that we were heading for a light, which I rightly presumed was their farmhouse. Eventually we ran aground, the two men got out, they pulled the boat a bit farther, and Jaap said, "You can get out now, Doctor."

The house and the adjacent shed apparently were situated on a knoll. Jaap had taken the boat around to the back of the house, where we were on the lee side. I waded through a foot of water to the back door. On either side, the water would probably be nearly up to my waist.

The farmer's wife said, "Oh, I am so glad you came, Doctor—the pain has eased off a little but she is still very ill." I was shown into a little bedroom where a young woman was lying. She told me she was seventeen years old, her periods were regular, the last one had been just a few days ago. During that afternoon she had been aware of a slight, dull ache in the belly, just like she used to have in the beginning of a period, but she had not paid much attention to it and it had gone away. She had had dinner, noticed nothing, and had gone to bed. Shortly after midnight she had awakened with a terrible pain. She immediately vomited but that did not relieve the pain.

The examination only confirmed my worst fears. Rigidity and tenderness on the abdominal wall, especially at one particular point—McBurney's.[1] I put the blanket back over her and told the mother, "She will have to have an operation—it's appendicitis." The mother and I went out into the

---

1. McBurney's point is located on the lower right abdomen between the umbilicus and the spine of the pelvic bone, where tenderness is present in appendicitis.

living room and I informed the men of the diagnosis. The father looked dubious: "You mean—she will have to go to the hospital, Doctor? For the operation?"

I knew that in the old days, until the beginning of the century, emergency procedures like cesarean sections and appendectomies were performed by general practitioners in rural areas on kitchen tables in out-of-the-way farmhouses. Even during World War II such interventions had been performed in the Netherlands under similar circumstances. However, I did not carry the necessary equipment for such heroic procedures in my bag. So I could only reply: "Yes, we must go to the hospital, and the sooner the better."

Everybody looked worried. The farmer cursed: "If only that damned telephone was workable!" Jaap was more practical: "What use would that be? There is nothing to be done but taking her to the dike in the boat and to Zevenbergen in the jeep. Then we will call our friend Herman and ask him to take us to Breda in the van."

The mother was fearful: "You mean to take her in the boat in this weather, sick as she is?" The father sighed. "I am afraid Jaap is right, Mother, it is the only thing we can do," then he turned to me and asked, "Is there really nothing you can do, Doctor?" I shook my head. "The only thing is an operation—if we would leave things as they are the appendix might perforate and then we'd have a really life-threatening situation. But have you got an icebag? Put ice in it and put it on her belly. It will relieve the pain a bit and probably slow down the progress of the inflammation."

Jaap piped in: "The boat will hold only three—certainly in this weather. Can you steer, Doctor?" I had done some sailing with a friend of mine in his boat and replied in the affirmative. He said, "I will row Maria and the Doctor across and take them to Zevenbergen."

The mother wrapped the girl in blankets, then Jaap lifted her up and carried her to the boat. The father followed with a tarpaulin. The two farmhands held the boat as Jaap gently laid his sister on the floor. The father covered her with the tarpaulin. The boat looked very small. Both Jaap and I sat with our legs spread, our feet each on one side of the girl on the bottom. Then the farmhands shoved us off.

Jaap informed me, "I left the lights of the jeep on. We will know we have rounded the house as soon as we can see them. You steer slightly to windward of it." The water was rather calm in the lee of the house, but coming out of it we got the full force of the storm. We were now going upwind and got the waves on our starboard bow. I saw the lights of the jeep and steered slightly to windward of it as Jaap had directed. We made very slow progress. Occasionally the girl moaned. Once we hit a particularly big wave which took us on the starboard bow and swept us some forty-five degrees off course. A gush of water came over us and the girl in the bottom of the boat shrieked. I had a vision of the Monday-morning newspapers carrying headlines like: "Young doctor drowned in effort to carry patient to safety."

When we touched bottom Jaap flung the line around a tree stump and knotted it. I told him to take a few minutes to catch his breath. Panting heavily, sweat pouring down his face, he nodded. Eventually saying, "I am all right now," he got out of the boat. He stood in ice-cold water which was up over his knees. As gently as he could he lifted his sister out of the boat and carried her up the dike. I went to the bow and jumped off. There the water was still ankle-deep but thanks to the Wellingtons I had been given I kept my feet dry.

We put Maria in the front seat, I got in the back, and Jaap took the wheel and started the engine. He managed to back the car on the narrow road and we drove back to Zevenbergen. "We'd better find out from the police if the road to Breda is still open," Jaap said. "What if it isn't?" I asked anxiously. Jaap replied, "The Breda police have a motorlaunch and in the army barracks in Breda they have amphibious vehicles." We went to the local police station, which had a black Land Rover parked in front of it.

Jaap went in and eventually came out with two police officers. One of them asked, "You are the doctor and this is the patient? We just came from Breda to find out how the situation is here. I suggest we take your patient back to Breda, to the General Hospital." I breathed a sigh of relief, got out, went into the station, and scribbled a note to the surgeon on duty.

In the meantime, the men had made the girl as comfortable as possible on the backseat of the Land Rover. Jaap wanted to return to the farm as soon as possible. He was trembling in his wet trousers. A local constable offered him a change of clothes.

I took the girl's hand and said: "You will be all right now, Maria." She brought my hand to her lips and kissed it. "I am glad you came in this beastly weather, Doctor—I am very grateful to you. God bless you."

"You must thank your brother," I told her, "I think he has saved your life."

She smiled at her brother and said, "Jaap, from now on I shall never quarrel with you again."

It was nearly seven o'clock when I got home. I phoned the hospital in Breda and spoke to the house surgeon to inform him about the patient who was on her way. He said he would have the theater prepared and remarked, "It must have been rather rough, going out in this weather?"

"You bet," I replied.

I switched on the radio for the early morning newscast. I learned that a combination of spring tide and a northwesterly gale had caused a number of dikes to collapse, and a state of emergency had been called for the provinces of Zeeland and Noord-Brabant in the southern Netherlands. It was the worst flood the country had known for centuries.

Later that morning the house surgeon phoned me to report that the girl had undergone an operation and a badly inflamed appendix had been removed. The girl was coming around in the recovery room. He praised my efforts at having gone out in the terrible weather. "Would you have done different?" I asked.

A few weeks later it turned out that about two thousand people in the Netherlands and Belgium had lost their lives in this disaster. But Jaap, the young farmer's son, through his courage and tenacity had saved at least one.

The Cardiac Event, the Doctor, and the Wife

Shmuel Reis
Galilee, Israel

The Cardiac Event

One February night in 1990, a fifty-five-year-old American, married, father of two and grandfather of one, a physicist in the computer industry, had a sudden collapse in the Ben-Gurion Airport, Israel. A few months earlier, he had had a medical examination, which had found no abnormality, and he wasn't taking any medication. The morning before his planned flight, he had a mild "stomach upset." At around midnight, waiting in the airport to board a jet to New York, he collapsed. While falling, he bumped his head against a heavy metal ashtray and lacerated the forehead so his face was covered with blood. A few bystanders rushed to his side, three of them physicians. He was turned on his back and when no breathing was detected, cardiopulmonary resuscitation (CPR) was administered.

Mouth-to-mouth breathing and closed chest massage were executed in the usual standard fashion. His pupils remained narrow, which encouraged the team to proceed for more than twenty-five minutes, even though there was no return of pulse or spontaneous breathing. By that time, the airport's defibrillator and standard emergency equipment were on hand. Appropriate medication was administered through an intravenous line, Ambu bag (a portable rubber mask and bladder) breathing was incorporated, and eventually three electric impulses to the chest were given. Forty minutes after the apparent cardiopulmonary arrest his heart resumed beating and spontaneous breathing returned; a few minutes later he was able to respond to his rescuers' commands by moving all four limbs. Fifty minutes after the beginning of the event, a mobile coronary care unit (CCU) arrived, took charge of the patient, and transferred him to a nearby hospital. A diagnosis of acute myocardial infarction was made and, following an uneventful recovery, he was discharged after ten days to a local cardiac rehabilitation facility from which he was allowed to fly back home ten days later. The patient was accompanied during the whole episode by his wife.

The Doctor

I was about to board a 747 jet to New York. One of my destinations was an Amelia Island meeting for "The Family in Family Medicine" conference, which I was to attend for the first time. I was doing last-minute shopping in the duty-free area when I noticed a man collapse to the ground, a small crowd gathering around him. Instinctively, I ran the thirty or so meters separating us and found myself leaning over a middle-aged man, his face covered with blood. I don't remember who did what exactly in the first few minutes. I recall turning him on his back, checking for breathing, and starting to do the motions of CPR. Another physician shared the ventilation and the chest massage work with me, while a third, an English-speaking woman, was on the patient's left side. Eventually she was the one to take care of establishing the intravenous line and medication administration. From time to time we checked his pupils, which stayed narrow. Although no pulse or spontaneous breathing was detected for at least twenty-five minutes, because the pupils kept staying narrow, we continued our work in an orderly manner. A paramedic joined us later, and we could upgrade our efforts; after three electric shocks, a sinus rhythm—a normal cardiac rhythm—was seen on the monitor, and spontaneous breathing resumed. I started talking to him, and he moved his arms and legs in response.

I remember the feeling of relief and joy that flooded me at that point. I washed my face and hands with some fluid from one of the intravenous bags lying around and watched the scene around me. The passengers were gone, since they had all boarded the jet. A few airport officials with walkie-talkies were standing around us; one reported that the airplane was still waiting for me and that a mobile CCU was on its way to us.

At the time I noticed a woman sitting a few meters away from us, watching the man on the marble floor. For some reason, it was evident she was the man's spouse. We started to exchange a few phrases. She gave me a brief history. She was calm and practical; I remember noticing how self-collected she was in these dramatic circumstances. I allowed myself to jokingly note my hope that her husband did not have AIDS. She responded appropriately with a smile saying: "If he did, I think I would have known it." Then she asked if she could sit next to him and talk to him, which she did; he responded very clearly. Meanwhile, the mobile CCU crew arrived. I handed the patient over to the physician who arrived and rushed over to the jet. I recall vividly walking to the aircraft's floor, tired (more than thirty minutes of CPR can be very tiring), shaking inside, with blood stains on my jeans.

During my tour of North America, a newspaper clipping reached me in Boston. An Israeli English-language daily had described briefly what took place at Ben-Gurion Airport a few weeks earlier.

Later on, I reached Amelia Island and enjoyed the company and conference. One day at lunch time, the telephone rang—the man who had collapsed at the airport was calling. In a deep, vibrant voice, he spoke about the night in the airport, hospital, recovery, and flying back home. He had managed somehow to track me down to express some of his feelings.

The Wife

Some time later I received a letter from the wife:

My husband and I celebrated our thirty-fifth wedding anniversary last week with our friends and family and we thought of you, Dr. Reis. Last month my son and daughter-in-law had their second daughter, and we thought of you. Every morning upon waking and finding my husband asleep next to me, I think of you. In the evening when I hear my husband's car door close, I think how lucky we were to be in an Israeli airport just at the right moment for you to have saved his life.

Not a day goes by that I don't relive those terrifying moments in the airport and my husband lying on the ground with a heart attack. It has become the most traumatic event in my life. It has certainly changed my comfortable assumption about life. I had noticed you in line earlier in the evening with your shopping cart filled with luggage waiting to clear customs. . . . I also noticed an attractive blond-haired woman in the purple striped knit outfit being detained at customs, who turned out to be Dr. Flaxie Flecther. Later, upon hearing the call for a doctor, the two of you would be working together to save my husband's life.

I must tell you of another incredible moment. When the call came for the two of you to board the plane, you were still administering CPR. Dr. Flecther came over to me and asked me if I was a religious person. I told her I hadn't thought about it, but I was spiritual. She told me to close my eyes and visualize my husband in the sun doing something he loves to do. She told me my strength would bring my husband back, and then she proceeded to pray to Jesus.

Just then the medics put the defibrillators on my husband again for the third time and he began to breathe on his own. How could we miss, you on the floor breathing life into my husband and the other doctor praying to Jesus. Now, tell me, does this happen very often to you? . . .

What were the possibilities of being at the right place at the right time for a trained person to administer CPR? In the whole universe, at that particular moment at that spot on earth my husband was saved by a total stranger.

The Kiss of Life

Ruth Bridgewater
Newcastle upon Tyne, United Kingdom

As the days grow autumnally shorter, and the week draws on, work winds its normal course through the eclectic humdrum life of the practice. The late call comes in as surgery is due to start: it's urgent, and it's only around the corner. Gladstone medical–bagged, drug and hassle-laden, I hasten round. Mrs. Smith is unwell. Let me be clearer: she has stopped breathing and is crumpled in her armchair, with only the gas fire to keep her warm. The house seems full of friends and relatives, rallying round, distressed at her plight. They cannot watch, they cannot leave, so they hover in the doorway.

And so to work. There is just barely room for her between the chair, the fire, and me. It's time to remember your ABC. A is for Airway—remove false upper teeth. B is for Breathing—absent. C is for Circulation—no pulse. Seizing control, I command her son to phone the ambulance (999 with blue lights and sirens blaring). It's time for resuscitation.

A precordial thump—a sharp blow to the sternum—and mouth-to-mouth yield no response. So, professionally, I get into the steady rhythm of mouth-to-mouth resuscitation and sternal compression—breaths, chest, breaths, chest. Nothing. The distress of the family rises

The cyclical nature of the working day is reassuring in its repetition: morning surgery, visits, evening surgery, visits. It's a common and predictable course, day in, day out, a tale of familiar patients with unremarkable stories. Why does the late call always come as surgery's about to start? I'm going to end up running late and being irritable, and the waiting patients will be cross. There's probably nothing wrong with her anyway.

But Mrs. Smith isn't well. She's arrested. This is a far cry from the cleanly white, clinically detached hospital world. I've nothing with me—not an airway, not suction, no monitor, nurse, anesthetist. Raw and exposed under the begging eyes of her relatives, I have no choice but to act. Now what to do first? A for Airway—she looks a bit like my gram without her teeth in. B—No, she's not breathing. C—I'm not going to be able to avoid this domestic resuscitation.

I hope my knights in the flashing white charger arrive soon. Mouth to mouth. Her lips are warm and soft, her face is smooth and downy. I'm kissing my nanna goodnight, but this is so much more intimate than a peck on the cheek. I'm trying to kiss Mrs. Smith back to life, like the Prince did to Sleeping Beauty. It's so intimate—too intimate. The paramedics arrive, and turn the physical closeness into clinical to hysterical proportions; luckily, the paramedics arrive. They have all the gear—the airway, the bag and mask, the defibrillator. Her airway becomes protected, her ventricular fibrillation is shocked. We can take an alive and breathing Mrs. Smith into hospital with us. We are met in the Accident and Emergency Department by the full crash team, who ooze efficiency. "So you claim she arrested, do you?"

detachment. I still smell the powder of her cheek on mine; I still sense the silkiness of the lips, and I touch mine to check how they feel.

A Story from a Sealed Room

Jeffrey M. Borkan
Southern Arava Valley, Negev, Israel

Some days you pack your black bag with antibiotics; other days you must fill it with antidotes to chemical warfare agents. I was told during my training that physicians are doomed to cynicism: although trained for great things, we encounter few opportunities for greatness but are buried in the mundane. However, during the 1991 Persian Gulf War, the challenges that I faced as a family physician in southern Israel stretched the usual boundaries. Since leaving a faculty position in family medicine at the University of Massachusetts in Worcester a few years ago, I have been the sole family physician of ten small kibbutzim (collective farming settlements) in an isolated region for the Negev desert on the Israeli–Jordanian border. My life during the war brought together the elements of medicine, community, and family that exemplify my role in this rural area.

During the night of January 16, 1991, we were informed of the start of military action against Iraq. We listened to the radio for hours. In the morning, the news analysts led us to believe that the war may have ended after a single night of bombing by the United States–led coalition. On January 17 all work was canceled throughout the country and an air of celebration reigned. We dozed off that night with a sense of peace.

But at 2:00 A.M. the spell was broken. I received a call from the husband of a woman for whom I was providing prenatal care. He excitedly told me that his wife had been having contractions since midnight and wondered if they should join us at our house. Since I generally see patients in their homes rather than mine, I asked why. He quickly explained that according to the radio news reports, Israel was under missile attack. The population had been instructed to enter their sealed rooms and put on gas masks.

The last hint of grogginess left me as the air raid sirens began to sound. I yelled to my wife to wake up our two small daughters and bring them into the room immediately. I told the caller to quickly bring his wife to my house and to bring their masks. Provisions, medicine, and emergency equipment were already in place. Time began to take on an unreal quality of expanding and contracting as we raced to finish preparing our sealed "shelter," which in this case was our bedroom. The couple arrived, already wearing their masks. The wife was pale with fear. Her eyes tearfully relayed her pain and anxiety. The husband and I hurriedly placed the final strips of nylon tape that were used to seal plastic sheeting over the doors and windows.

I assisted my wife in placing our screaming six-month-old daughter into her plastic "anti-gas" tent and secured a gas mask hood over our whimpering four-year-old child's face. Our hearts ached as we did this. To what harm, both physical and psychological, were we exposing our children? Why were we, their parents, exposing them to these frightful protective measures, the terror of war, and the risk of death?

The initial tasks were completed within ten minutes. The small room was filled with crying and fear. I struggled to assess the situation and reestablish calm, but on this, the first night of attack, it was difficult to estimate the risk since so little was known of the Iraqi threat. Were we one of the intended targets? Was this a conventional or nonconventional missile attack? Would the missiles be followed by Iraqi or Jordanian planes or troops?

Eventually we were able to calm the children. The visiting couple took their positions at the head of our bed, timing contractions between radio an nouncements from civil defense. I huddled with my wife at the foot of the bed, surveying the scene. What were my priorities here, attending to my patient or my family? I struggled to do both, leaving the question for later.

After some delay, we were informed by the chief army spokesman that missiles had fallen in several areas and that there were multiple casualties. We were asked to stay in our sealed rooms, but gas masks could come off and the children could be removed from their plastic tents.

As the hours passed into morning and the sun rose behind the sealed windows, I periodically checked my patient's progress and monitored the fetal heart rate by Doppler ultrasound. The woman progressed quickly, and I became concerned that she would soon give birth on our bed with our children in attendance. The emergency medical system was still paralyzed, and transport could not be arranged. Searching through our bedroom closets and through the emergency equipment I had stored, I assembled enough implements for a birth, including suction and local anesthetics.

As the woman reached transition, the point at which she is ready to push the baby out, the radio announced that all missiles had been armed with conventional warheads and that everyone could leave their houses. We then received telephone permission to travel out of the settlement in an ambulance. I quickly prepared the patient for transport, and we began the forty-minute trip to the hospital. I felt an eerie "end of the world" sensation as we drove down deserted highways and into a shuttered city with no one on the streets. Soon after arrival at the hospital, my patient gave birth to a healthy baby girl. New life emerged out of a night of death and terror; hope remained.

The Knock on the Door at Night

Bob Stever

Kratie, Cambodia

From 1962 to 1964, my wife Ann and I lived in Cambodia where I volunteered as a physician for CARE–MEDICO[2] in a remote section of northeast Cambodia called Kratie (now Krâchéh). At the time all the physicians in the country worked in the capital city except the four physicians in our clinic and two others at Lompat in the mountains near Vietnam. Health care was organized by a "Médecin-en-chef," with one paramedical person assigned to each province to oversee total health care in that area.

During our stay I gradually became aware that we were on one of many routes of the Ho Chi Minh Trail that followed a dirt highway only kilometers from Vietnam and paralleled the border north to Laos, thus connecting Hanoi with Saigon. The fighting had already begun in Vietnam; we were not only uneasy at the proximity, but saddened that there was war.

Ann kept all the accounts for the clinic and filled in where she was needed while I plunged into the clinic with hundreds of patients to be seen between eight and one o'clock. Then the heat became too intense for any creature not reptilian. An internist joined me in the clinic and a surgeon operated in the modern, green-tiled, air-conditioned operating room that had been donated by the organization.

Each morning patients gathered outside the clinic. People came from everywhere: some motored up the Mekong River on a commercial river boat, some came from the local town, Kratie, and some, who were of a different racial and language group from the Cambodians, came from the hills. Hunkering quietly for hours until the clinic opened, those waiting helped the ill and led us to the sickest ones when the morning triage began. No one pushed ahead. Instead, they shared news with one another from distant parts of the country. For some, a visit to the clinic was a social event.

Highlanders, the Khmai Loer (Loer meaning high), were claimed by Cambodia, though these tribes never belonged to any country. Thousands of these tiny groups occupy the high mountains along the Himalayan chain from Tibet, China, and Burma to Laos, Vietnam, and Cambodia. They had been pushed into the hills centuries or even millennia before by waves of invaders from Indonesia, India, and Thailand, and spoke little Cambodian (Khmer). They struck me as gentle, perceptive, and wise. Their stocky, powerful bodies,

---

2. CARE (Cooperative for American Relief, Inc.) is a worldwide charity founded in 1945; in 1962 MEDICO (Medical International Cooperation Organization), a medical relief agency, became part of it.

prominent wide cheekbones, round eyes, mahogany skin, and straight, jet-black hair reminded me of Polynesians.

The men wore narrow loincloths, sometimes a shirt if it was cool, but seldom any shoes. Thick ivory plugs pierced their ears, and they usually chomped on a homemade cigar. Over their shoulders they slung their poison-tipped darts with a tiny powerful bow made of hardwood. Always present, they were ready for hunting or protection and formed part of the dress code. The women wrapped around their waists long sarongs, hand-woven from a tough cotton with red and black horizontal stripes.

One stormy monsoon night I was startled awake by banging on the louvered French doors of the clinic below. Lying in bed half awake, I had visions of the Vietcong arriving to raid the clinic or even kidnap us. The banging changed to a threatening rattle of the doors as if someone were trying to break them open.

Cambodian people were afraid of "evil spirits" at night, so they never ventured out late. Who could it be? With no choice but to answer the door, I threw on some clothes and descended the great stairs to the red tile foyer of the French colonial house. Full of curiosity, yet also some fear, I lit all the lights, unbolted the double French doors, and flung them both open expecting to see the Vietcong army.

There on the steps stood a Khmai Loer couple holding a critically ill baby. The Khmai Loer are not afraid of the dark, so they had walked two days to the clinic, arriving in the wee hours of the morning. For a long moment we stared at each other, squinting in the bright lights of the clinic. Though I spoke some Cambodian, they did not. The moment was awkward as we strained to communicate.

Suddenly the baby boy in the woman's arms, already with labored breathing, gasped, rattled, and stopped breathing. The mother thrust him into my arms. Several squeezes of the tiny chest between my hands restored his breathing, only to have it stop again, but he responded each time to further squeezes. I indicated they should follow me as I dashed for the operating room where there was oxygen, medicine, and intravenous fluids. It was incredible to me that they had arrived just at the moment when the baby approached death.

Entering the surgical suite, they must have been overwhelmed by the modern, green-tiled room with its air-conditioning and surgical lights, all out of character with the surrounding jungle. But after one sweeping look, they focused their complete attention on the baby and me. The four of us were alone in the suite. All the nurses and personnel had left for the day at 1:30 P.M.

Quickly the couple understood through my gestures what I wanted them to do, never failing for one second to follow my instructions. The father held the oxygen mask over the baby's face while the mother supported the baby's arm so I could start intravenous fluids and antibiotics. They had never seen oxygen hiss through a mask or fluids poked into an arm, but they never questioned me, not even with a glance. It is always difficult to find a tiny vein in a baby's arm, and while I searched, there were several respiratory arrests. But the father now knew how to pump the chest.

Finally the baby stabilized, as his pneumonia and dehydration responded to the oxygen and fluids. His breathing, now continuous, had no further arrests. The parents' adept assistance had made the difference. The pneumonia resolved promptly, to the relief of all. Every day in the hospital for the next two weeks, I was met with a grin from the parents, and even, it seemed, from the baby.

On their departure day, they came to the clinic to thank me. The mother reached into a small hand-woven purse slung over her shoulder, extracted a tiger's claw, pressed it to my hand, and closed my fingers over it. A tiger's claw represented such good luck in Cambodia that no one would part with one easily.

With a lump in my throat, I watched them begin their two-day trek to the hills, thankful that I had not delayed answering the door.

References

Downie, R. S. 1994. *The Healing Arts*. Oxford: Oxford University Press.

Hart, J. T. 1988. *A New Kind of Doctor*. London: Merlin Press.

Keay, J., and J. Keay, eds. 1994. *Collins Encyclopaedia of Scotland*. London: Harper-Collins.

Shorter, E. 1985. *Bedside Manners*. New York: Simon and Schuster.

White, K. L. 1988. *The Task of Medicine: Dialogue at Wickenburg*. Menlo Park, Calif.: Henry J. Kaiser Family Foundation.

Suffering and Shame

Reflections

Howard F. Stein

The four stories in this chapter illustrate exquisitely the close kinship of suffering and shame—for patient, doctor, family, community, and health care institution alike. The experience of suffering—say, in an illness episode—often triggers a powerful sense of shame as well as guilt. The experience of shame often triggers profound suffering. Shame can be a fleeting feeling, keen or vague; an unconscious emotion; and even a central organizing principle of personal life (taking the form, for instance, of the pursuit of honor, of pride, of vengeance, of withdrawal, of hiding).

Shame can be one's response to the inner self (which includes and condenses mental representations of emotionally significant people and those of oneself) or to public humiliation (Lynd 1958; Erikson 1963; Lansky 1994). Its source, or at least its current referent, can be internal or external (Tangney et al. 1996). Shame is triggered when one feels a terrible discrepancy between who one imagines, wishes, or expects oneself to be, and how, suddenly, one in fact is, private or public. Two ways of seeing oneself, or of hearing oneself, or of being seen and heard by others are irreconcilable. Shame—and the effort to recover from shame—attempts to fill the gap. It is little wonder that murderers, because of shame, often take out the eyes and cut off the ears of their victims (Gilligan 1996).

The sense of shame can be incapacitating, paralyzing. Alternately, it can be liberating, perhaps by bringing to light facets of oneself of which one had been unaware (as if to say, "That's me too!"). The experience of shame in families and workplaces can lead to violent acts of retaliation (Gilligan 1996; Diamond 1997). Finally, the sequential triad of interpersonal conflict, shame, and blame can regulate and even ruin a physician–patient relationship (Martin 1993).

Shame, like its kin guilt, is a court of judgment, stern in condemnation: simplistically, *guilt* for something one has *done; shame* for something one *is*. The two are emphases, not absolutes. One can suffer moral masochism for either, or for both. Ostensibly "shame" cultures are rife with "guilt," as De Vos (1973) described for Japan. Conversely, I can be ashamed of something I *did,* because what I did reflects poorly on who and what I am, on what I think of myself, and on what others think of me. One can feel both guilt and shame for the same deed, and in the same situation.

Developmentally speaking, both emotions in adulthood live in the shadow of childhood's anxious world of giants and dwarfs, of real and imagined immensity and smallness (Kilborne 1995). All current experiences of shaming and of shame involve some magnitude of transference—projection in the widest sense—from childhood situations and their inner elaborations onto real contemporary events and relationships.

The stories in this chapter remind me how central, rather than peripheral, so-called psychosocial facets of illness are. In the third story, for instance, with the Iranian-general-now-humble shopkeeper, secret shame is clearly pathogenic, that is, part of the cause of his chest pain, his "physical" suffering. Does he not truly ache in the symbolic heart, even if his physician helps him to accept that he does not have life-threatening cardiovascular disease? Part of his suffering, successor to his shame, is that his life-meaning, his identity, has been threatened—as lethal as any organic disease.

The stories in this chapter remind me that the "foreign" is less a place than a state of mind. "Foreign" is a place in thought we do not yet include inside ourselves. A well-told story ultimately turns geography partly into fiction: suddenly, *there* could be *here.* The foreign is the familiar not yet realized. To understand a good story is to universalize its sense of place. It begins with an experience somewhere, and ends with an experience that in essence could be anywhere. It is less strange because we are less estranged from some once-new part of ourselves. We suddenly realize that, despite the alienness of the address, "This could happen here," or "I have seen something like that right here." The harrowing tale from the Ivory Coast could be a story from a rural patient's search for care in the urban United States; or it could be the story of an inner-city ambulance rushing from hospital to hospital, no hospital willing to give a nonpaying patient sanctuary. It is not that locale and local context are irrelevant, but in the hands of a good storyteller, they become comprehensible as universal issues. They are no longer exotic tales.

The bridge or wall between foreign and familiar also is the bridge or wall between the patient's shame and the physician's shame (or the teaching doctor and the resident's, triggered by the patient's). Shame can be a trigger for flight and defense, or for empathy and insight. The difference between these is nothing less than the inability and ability to listen, the inability and ability to heal, respectively. We understand another's shame through access to our own; and only with that access can we help another person.

The stories in this chapter come from day-to-day family practice sources, not from medical rarities: from their responsibilities with emergency medicine, from obstetrical/gynecological practice, from ordering and interpreting tests, from dealing with such vague and diffuse patient complaints as chest pain, from life crisis, from telephone medicine, and from the experiences of abandonment. For doctor and patient alike, the linked lives of suffering and shame are not at all foreign and rare. The challenge for the practitioner is whether we can bear our own shame and suffering and be able to hear, to see, to feel—and to respond from the uncomfortable knowledge (Stein 1988) these provide us.

The culture(s) of biomedicine have a constellation of values, attitudes, beliefs, and expectations—all of which become incorporated as part of practitioners' defensive structures—that tend to make it difficult to hear and respond compassionately to patients' shame (Stein 1985, 1990; Stein and Apprey 1990). At the same time, this "constellation" tends to place physicians at considerable risk for attacks of shame and guilt. Here I refer to the wish to be in control and the expectation that the clinician should be in control, the belief that one is a failure if one cannot control the disease or the patient, the expectation that one will be able to cure the patient or at least persuade the patient to "comply" with medical advice, and so on.

Physicians, not only patients, often live out a hidden narrative structure or story line of how assessment, diagnosis, and treatment should unfold. When the expected sequence of the story does not materialize, or the ending is not what it "should" be, the physician frequently feels ashamed or guilty, self-blaming; alternatively, the physician projects these feelings onto the patients, becoming angry, distant, ridiculing, even abusive. The "wrong" clinical outcome often feels like professional and personal failure. In the first story in this chapter, the physician's sense of shame at the end would seem in part to be an example of this disparity between the expected, wished-for, ending and the ending that really takes place.

All four stories should be recognizable in the reader's own life, translatable, that is, from the writer's idiom to the reader's. "There" is less strange or exotic than we think, or compel it to be. "Strange" is inseparable from the conscious or unconscious act of "estrangement." Distance must be measured in distancing, not only in meters or miles. Here we must confront our own potential shame and defenses against it in their role of making the potentially familiar into the alien. *What if* "there" were "here"? What would we be? What would we feel? The stories in this chapter were, each in a different way, painful to read. It must be that way. Whether we be reader, doctor, or patient, we can comprehend suffering only by suffering ourselves (*com*-passion derives from that sense of suffering *with*). That is, in each instance of successful storytelling or successful doctoring, "there" becomes "here."

In the first story, the Ivory Coast is not so far from Oklahoma or New York City as it may seem. Themes of poverty, isolation, disease, suffering, waiting, gratitude, and shame are interwoven. The patient is profoundly and expressively grateful for what the doctor did for him. At the same time, the physician feels a sharp pang of shame for the yawning gaps between what he was able to do for his patient, what he wished (maybe even expected) he could have done for his patient, and his patient's deep gratitude. It was as if the physician were saying, through his shame: "How can you be grateful for so much, when I have been able to do so little for you?" The old theory of "relative deprivation" would seem to be at work here.

A good story confirms experience and gives new experience—and a new way of experiencing. A good story should help us to heal. It should make for us more room in our inner spaces. This one does. As I read the story of a patient shuttled by taxi from his village to the government hospital, then to the mission hospital, I kept thinking of similar gaps in compassion between rural and urban medicine in the United States, and of how, in many cities I know of, patients are desperately shuttled by ambulance from hospital to hospital in search of a place of sanctuary for "the medically indigent," which is to say, the unwanted, nonpaying, uninsured patients. Further, distance, isolation, and strangerhood are universal players in the drama of rural and urban medicines. The story reminds us how important relatives are in clinical decision making (including decisions to stay or leave), and how language everywhere closes or widens distance. Finally, the story shows how a physician's decision to take clinical responsibility can begin to break the vicious cycles of hopelessness and exploitability experienced by patients.

In the second story, the doctor finds herself "caught" by a pregnant patient in the act of thinking of herself rather than of the patient. When physicians order medical tests, who benefits? Often the test treats the physician's own anxiety over current or anticipated shame (Stein 1985). Shame and guilt alike can be used to fend off deep grief. In this story in which an anencephalic fetus is eventually born dead, the sense of shame lies in the physician's recognition of the wide disparity between what and whom she felt she should have been thinking about and what and whom she had in fact placed first in importance. Both patient and doctor worried that they had done something wrong: the mother, an act of commission, the physician, an act of omission, specifically, failure to order a screening blood test sooner. Sometimes—insidiously—the doctor (specifically, the doctor's anxiety) becomes the second patient in treatment in the effort to undo his or her own sense of shame. And sometimes, as in this story, what the patient needs to talk about and what the doctor needs to talk about collide rather than coincide.

Along the way in this second story, an act of grace occurs, one that made "doing" and "controlling" less important. Saving face and ordering tests became less important than her relationship with the patient. Even medical knowledge becomes an often magical form of control. It is as if to say: "Somehow, if I just knew, or knew earlier, what was wrong, I could have fixed it and it could have turned out right." The patient reminds her doctor of the pathos beyond the quest for control: even if they had known what was wrong, the mother would not have been able to keep the baby. The flight toward control is often a flight from feeling.

Feeling shame (and probably remorse), the doctor in this second story did not try to flee into action or haughty moralism, but learned from her feelings to attend more closely to the patient's concerns. She truly listened to her patient's near-whispered protest. The moment of shame became the birth of compassion. Being with the patient at a crucial moment became the most important "clinical task." The story is truly one of grace.

The third story introduces a common triad: the patient, a medical trainee or apprentice, and a faculty physician. Here, when the resident "presented" or reported a summary of his medical findings and treatment plan to his supervisor, the faculty physician decided to talk with the patient herself. In the third story, the patient's unexplained, mysterious chest pain, together with its timing, becomes the bearer of a secret—one literally embodied—story of shame in an immigrant. The author's writing is as beautiful to the reader as the gift of listening must have been liberating to the patient. The patient's inner storm is hauntingly sandwiched by the author's anticipation of the approaching winter storm outside. The storm metaphor becomes almost unbearable as I hear the physician inquire into the timing of the symptoms in this Iranian expatriate: could there be any connections with the then-current Middle Eastern war between Iraq and the United States, the U.S.-named Operation Desert Storm? In the midst of so much emotional and physical debris, the physician sat still, listened, probed, and listened more. Clinically, the story of the liberation from shame's suffering is the grace of someone who stays put and cares to hear the story out. Biomedically, the time taken by the faculty physician to listen to the patient's story also reaps dividends in saving time and money for unnecessary tests that would have been done instead of listening.

There are also profound lessons about language, subtler than in the first story, but pointed. The resident had asked the patient about issues of "stress" in his life, and the patient replied there were none. The patient's secret shame had to be elicited more indirectly than the code word "stress" to which we give far too much weight!

The fourth story begins as a tactful if exasperating exchange in telephone medicine, it ends with a jarring understanding of the flight into madness as a flight from the shame of public abandonment at so private and collective a moment in life as one's marriage. Even the patient's rewriting of reality—called "paranoiac delusion psychosis" by the medical profession—makes sense as something *we* ourselves could do, not only *those* from whom we diagnostically differentiate ourselves by calling *them* insane (Devereux 1980). Her delusion was her private, if pathetic, recovery from mortification by shame. In her madness, she was still beloved; she turned her rage into a persecution fantasy. She becomes to us less alien and more imaginable. It is as if the reader might say: "Maybe if that had happened to me and I felt that bad, I could have reacted that way, too."

Taken together, these four brief stories offer unexpected wealth in understanding the interior of suffering and shame. In all of them, there is no "there" that could not be, in recognizable form, "here" as well.

The Reluctant Samaritan

Kami Kandola
Ivory Coast

It was late Friday night when the taxi pulled up to the mission hospital. In the back seat, a young Ivoirian farmer lay motionless. His grossly deformed right arm was hot and swollen with purulent discharge oozing from a sutured wound. He was unable to walk. Another man (presumably a relative) quickly exited from the car holding X-rays. "A tree fell on him two days ago," was the fragmented French translation of his native Lobi.

The story then unfolded. Several days ago, while chopping a tree, this unfortunate man had misjudged the direction of its fall, sustaining the impact on his right forearm and hip. He was carried to the nearest dispensary where the nurse sutured the gaping wound on his wrist and attempted to transfer him to the nearest hospital, after charging CFA Fr60,000 (1 French franc = 100 Ivoirian (CFA) francs, a cost of approximately $100 [U.S. 1997]). After a wait of one and a half days, a taxi arrived at the relatively isolated village. The patient, who of course, had no access to a painkiller, then endured a grueling six-hour drive on unpaved roads half washed away by recent rain.

Upon arrival at the government hospital, the patient was admitted only after paying an exorbitant fee and after a radiographic analysis of the extent of his injuries was obtained. The patient lay on his hospital cot for hours without having received a diagnosis or even basic antiseptic care. No one from the hospital staff visited him. Frustrated by the lack of medical attention, relatives discharged him from the hospital and brought him to the mission compound.

I was not the doctor on duty, but a quick perusal of the X-rays revealed several serious breaks of his right forearm and right hip, including a transverse severely angulated radial and ulnar fracture of the mid-forearm and a spiral, displaced fracture of the right femur. The prognosis appeared bleak. All the specialized orthopedic facilities were to be found in the city (another ten-hour drive), and again the service fees were prohibitive. If the patient was ever to walk normally again, an open reduction and internal fixation of his femur would be required. In addition, he suffered the infectious consequences of an open fracture of his right forearm, which had been mistakenly sutured closed.

What a dilemma! Lack of orthopedic skills as well as anesthesiologist at the mission hospital would provide the patient no advantage in regaining the function of his limbs. The nurse on duty took a simple approach. "Send him back to the government hospital. We can't help him here." This pessimistic response could seal the patient's fate.

"No," I replied. "Let's call the doctor on duty."

Suboptimal care was better than no care at all, so the patient was admitted. His right arm required amputation when the overwhelming infection responded poorly to broad-spectrum antibiotics. His right femoral fracture was externally fixated and put into traction.

I left the hospital several weeks later. My last memory of the patient was embedded in my mind. His right leg was hooked up to the ceiling by ropes and pulleys as he waved goodbye with his right arm stump. His eyes reflected a deep gratitude. "God bless you! I can never thank you enough for what you have done for me."

For some reason, I felt ashamed.

Grace

Mindy Smith
Chelsea, Michigan

Her name is Mary. She is a bit shy and soft-spoken, with intelligent gray eyes and a wonderful, warm laugh. I was present for the birth of her two boys, both emerging with the vitality and lusty cry that dissipates the last bit of anxiety that we share with our patients just before a baby's arrival. This third pregnancy seemed to be going well, although I often found Mary hard to read as we reviewed the past months' progress and she asked her few pointed questions.

While I was away, shortly before week 24 of her pregnancy, Mary saw my partner for a routine visit. She expressed concern that something didn't feel right. She had been reading through her patient education materials and wondered if she could have the alpha-fetoprotein test[1] performed. He informed her that it was really too late in the pregnancy for this test and that her risk was low, because of her negative family history. He offered to perform an ultrasound if she was still concerned. She agreed to proceed with the ultrasound that Thursday afternoon.

Having never diagnosed anencephaly,[2] my partner was afraid to make this diagnosis based on his in-office sonogram. Instead, he told Mary something did appear to be wrong with the baby, but that he was uncertain and needed to refer her to the university sonographers. An appointment was scheduled for the following Monday. I returned that evening and found his message on my machine. I was horrified. I had no idea whether I had told her about the test and if so, doubted that I had documented our conversation. I worried that I might be facing my first lawsuit for missed diagnosis; in addition, I had created a situation with no easy recourse for Mary compared with an early second trimester abortion had the test been positive. I anguished about her pain and knew that we couldn't wait until Monday.

I arranged through my contact in the radiology department to proceed with the ultrasound the next day and called Mary that night. I explained that my partner had left a message and I didn't want her to worry over the weekend. She seemed grateful but declined my offer to be present for the test, as she doubted that anything was seriously wrong. I went anyway.

The radiologist confirmed what my partner had feared. The boy she carried had anencephaly. I went into the room to tell her the diagnosis, preparing

1. The alpha-fetoprotein test is a screening blood test used early in pregnancy to detect spinal cord abnormalities and Down's syndrome.
2. Anencephaly refers to major defects in the development of the the brain and the bones of the cranial vault, often with the absence of cerebral and cerebellar hemispheres.

myself for her anger and questions. As she wept, I held her. When she could finally speak, her first question surprised me. "What did I do wrong?"

"My God," I said, "you didn't do anything wrong. These are accidents of nature. We can only grieve, and then, if you want, I will help you decide what to do." I paused and went on, "I only wish that I had performed the blood test so that we could have known sooner. . . ." My voice trailed off.

Her answer was so quick that it took me by surprise. "What would that have changed?" she said, her voice almost a whisper, "'I don't get to keep him anyway." I felt so ashamed that I had given a single thought to my own interests and so grateful that I could be with her at that moment.

I offered to drive her home. We spoke little and I arranged to meet with her and her husband as soon as they felt able to talk. At that meeting a few days later, we made plans to induce labor. I showed them pictures of what their child would look like and we discussed how to approach the boys with the news that their brother would not be coming home. Mary decided to write a letter from the baby to the boys explaining why he couldn't be with them, and she planned to create an album as a remembrance.

The delivery went as well as could be expected. She bore it with a grace that humbled me. I wept with them as she held her stillborn son Jack, uncovering his head so that she could see and touch all of him. "Look at his beautiful hands," she remarked, "and his small and perfect toes." We took pictures and footprints for the album. Jack's body was sent to pathology and Mary and her husband made the long trip home.

Newfound Lands

Ann C. Macaulay
Montreal, Quebec

It was the end of the day, a cold day in February 1991, in the midst of a major winter snowstorm. I was the staff physician in the Family Medicine Teaching Unit of a Montreal hospital associated with McGill University.

A first-year resident wanted to discuss a sixty-year-old patient who had come in with chest pain. The resident presented his history and physical examination. The patient had immigrated to Canada from Iran, and his past medical history, current history, and examination were negative. The resident had diagnosed chest pain secondary to musculoskeletal causes and felt comfortable in sending him home and offering him a return appointment. I inquired if there were any issues of stress. The resident, a competent one, stated he had asked those questions but the patient had answered "No."

I decided to see the patient myself to ensure that the diagnosis and management were correct. I entered the small, bleak examining room and noticed that the snow was still falling heavily. I inwardly hoped I would be able to leave the hospital before the storm closed any roads.

The patient was attractive and well dressed. I asked a few standard questions, verifying exactly what the resident had described to me, but somehow I felt something was missing. I then asked him how long he had been in Canada and what his occupation was. He replied he had immigrated ten years ago and was minding a small store. I was surprised, since he gave me the impression that he had a high level of education and good executive skills. Probing for the missing detail, I asked his occupation in Iran before he immigrated to Canada. He quietly answered that he had been one of the highest ranking generals in the Iranian army under the Shah and had been forced to leave Iran with the coming of the Ayatollah. In a very direct question, I asked him if the current Gulf War was bothering him. For a moment, I thought he would cry, but he started to talk.

His story was about his defeat and capture by the Ayatollah's army, followed by solitary confinement and torture. He described being kept for weeks in a cell that was too small to allow him to lie down. He also spoke of the deaths of many of his soldiers and some family members and how he felt responsible for so much loss of life. His escape had been difficult and he had been unable to settle into any suitable work in Montreal. Since the beginning of the current Gulf War, he had experienced intense pains in different parts of his body together with significant sleep disturbances and severe nightmares. So, we sat and talked. He easily accepted the link between the mind and the body and was comforted to hear that his chest pain resulted from his current tensions. He declined the offer for a follow-up visit.

The depth of snow and impending closure of the roads no longer seemed important. If necessary, I could find a bed in the hospital. After the patient had left, the resident and I talked and we realized that the unit was currently seeing a higher number of Iranians than usual. We reflected that these patients had left Iran for a safe new home without realizing that the pain of their own country's past would follow to their newfound lands.

Beyond the Lock

Hans Antonneau
Berchem, Belgium

"I can't take it, I must call him," she thought.

She couldn't hold out too long before she heard the voice that each time brought her such comforting rest. Finally, she lifted the telephone and called the familiar number. "Hello, Doctor," she said hopefully, "will I be safe?"

"Yes, Simonne," he said sleepily. "I'm sure that you will be safe. But don't you know how late it is?" To himself, he said, "It's two o'clock in the morning, dammit."

"Oh, I'm sorry, Doctor, but are you certain?"

"Yes, yes. Go to sleep now, I am certain that nothing will happen to you. Believe me—you can sleep. You'll see tomorrow that nothing will have happened."

"Thank you. Good-bye, Doctor."

"Goodnight, Simonne."

She turned out the light and lay in her bed, eyes wide open, listening to the sounds that plagued her from above the ceiling. It had been two years since that man moved in upstairs with the sole purpose to end her life.

"I probably shouldn't have bothered the doctor this time," she thought. "It was quiet today." The whole evening Simonne had heard nothing. Not even the soft shuffling of his feet across the floorboards. "I would rather hear steps in the kitchen now and then, or the water tap running in the bathroom," she thought. "Then at least I will know what he's up to."

She had taken a peek around his vacant apartment before he came to live there. It was just like hers. There was a large living room at the front with a small kitchen next to it. In the small entry she saw four doors: one each for the bedroom, the bathroom, the closet, and the smaller, extra room. More than anything it was this last one that brought her anxiety. She was sure that it was in this small room, just above her ironing room, that he spent his time conjuring up his plans to one day bring a gruesome end to her life. She was convinced that the fateful day would soon be dawning. Still, she dared to harbor a faint hope that it wasn't yet that far along. When she knew for sure that he was in the kitchen or the living room, she could rest a little easier.

When he was cooking or reading the newspaper, he would hardly be able to focus on his scheming to bring about her demise. She knew exactly when he ate, what TV programs he watched, and when he went to bed. From the sounds she was able to make out from the toilet, she even thought she had a good notion of his daily habits there. She would be fine until she heard him

46

on the telephone or receiving a visitor. An episode of this sort would raise her anxiety level several times over. "What does a man who lives alone have to say to anyone?" she thought. "I live alone too and I've not yet experienced anything that I couldn't finish telling about in a few minutes!"

She had little doubt that all those lengthy conversations were about her. He had surely located a co-conspirator to assist him with the murder.

Now she remembered. Tonight she had called the doctor not because the man upstairs was mulling around in the small room, and not because he sat plotting with his co-conspirator, but because it was Thursday. Every Thursday evening, without exception, he watched his favorite TV program. Tonight she heard nothing.

"The doctor was right," she thought. "I am safe because it's already late into the night. I must have fallen asleep just now when I took that pill at seven o'clock! Yes! I remember. He was in the small room. The doctor was right."

Quietly she lay there recalling the first time she saw him on the stairs two years before. He was the exact image of Herman, but twenty-eight years older. Herman had grown older, his mustache didn't give him that friendly walruslike appearance from those earlier days. It was thinner now, a gray stripe under a much-too-sharp nose. Little by little she became convinced that the graying man upstairs with the mustache was really Herman.

At first she was happy. He had come back to find her again. Maybe he wanted to make everything right. Yet she couldn't understand why he only nodded curtly when they met in the hall. What was worse, after a while he acted as if she wasn't there. No matter what she would do to attract his attention by wearing a sheer gown, waiting for him to walk by her door, it didn't seem to affect him. It was at that point that she understood that he wanted to kill her to erase his feeling of guilt. She knew Herman. "He doesn't want me to live any longer in the hell for which he is to blame. Herman has come to liberate me," she decided.

With the consistency of the tides, the image returned to her of that horrible day. She once again remembered that fateful moment, twenty-eight years ago, when Herman left her standing at the altar on their wedding day. She relived it as though it were yesterday.

He had stepped out of the car that brought them to the church and just walked away, past her friends and family, and past the lock of the canal where she had enjoyed the happiest moments of her young life.

Epilogue

The eventful moment at the lock on Simonne's wedding day effectively brought an end to her life, as she had known it. Simonne is now living in the geriatric department of the psychiatric hospital of her village. She was unable to withstand the continuous delusional thoughts and interpsychic pressures which emanated from the belief that her old lover was living in the apartment above her. Perhaps what we doctors call "paranoiac delusion psychosis" is just another way of looking at the world.

References

Devereux, G. 1980. *Basic Problems of Ethno-Psychiatry.* Chicago: University of Chicago Press.

De Vos, G. A. 1973. *Socialization for Achievement.* Berkeley: University of California Press.

Diamond, M. A. 1997. Administrative assault: a contemporary psychoanalytic view of violence and aggression in the workplace. *American Review of Public Administration* 27(3):228–47.

Erikson, E. H. 1963. *Childhood and Society.* Rev. ed. New York: Norton.

Gilligan, J. 1996. *Violence: Our Deadly Epidemic and Its Causes.* New York: Grosset/Putnam.

Kilborne, B. 1995. Of creatures large and small: size anxiety, psychic size, shame, and the analytic situation. *Psychoanalytic Quarterly* 64(4):672–90.

Lansky, M. R. 1994. Shame: contemporary psychoanalytic perspectives. *Journal of the American Academy of Psychoanalysis* 22(3):433–41.

Lynd, H. M. 1958. *On Shame and the Search for Identity.* New York: Science Editions.

Martin, J. T. 1993. Shame and the origin of physician–patient conflict. *Journal of the American Osteopathic Association* 93(4):486, 489–91.

Stein, H. F. 1985. *The Psychodynamics of Medical Practice.* Berkeley: University of California Press.

Stein, H. F. 1988. Uncomfortable knowledge: an ethnographic clinical training model. *Family Systems Medicine* 6(1):117–28.

Stein, H. F. 1990. *American Medicine as Culture.* Boulder, Colo.: Westview Press.

Stein, H. F., and M. Apprey. 1990. *Clinical Stories and Their Translations.* Charlottesville: University Press of Virginia.

Tangney, J. R. P., S. Miller, L. Flicker, and D. H. Barlow. 1996. Are shame, guilt, and embarrassment distinct emotions? *Journal of Personality and Social Psychology* 70(6):1256–69.

Learning from Patients

Reflections

Jack H. Medalie

What is the most effective way to learn to become a physician, a healer? How can health care providers maintain and enhance competence throughout their careers? Textbooks, lectures, journal clubs to discuss new articles, research, Internet surfing, or tele-education? They all "contribute greatly to the life-long learning of medicine, but they are not a substitute for patients" (Melni-koff 1989).

This chapter is a powerful illustration of the multiple ways patients teach. Patients, no doubt, "define the course of medicine: their disease mani-festations, if unusual, challenge dogma and can lead to reflection and change"(Anon 1994). Every physician remembers certain patients, their "ill-ness scripts," and presentations etched permanently into their memories more vividly than any textbook description. As Dubb (1983) has written, "Learn-ing in medicine is not merely the acquisition of more facts. Nor is teaching confined to our colleagues and seniors. Each of us is both a student and a teacher. Furthermore, much of our learning, and hopefully WISDOM, may be derived from patients."

However, patients do not merely provide the palate for clinical patho-physiology or disease management. There are lessons that go beyond the cog-nitive, that touch the other side of doctoring, the inner cord. It is not only the "Patients Who Changed My Practice," as in the series published in the *British Medical Journal,* but also the "patients who transformed me."

For many decades clinical educators have taught the importance of the medical history. Peabody in Boston, Osler in Baltimore and London, and Forman in Cape Town are examples of clinicians who showed that a good medical history was the key to a correct medical diagnosis. In the 1950s, Richardson and Ackerman (both in New York) demonstrated the importance of the family history to the individual patient. During the same period, Balint in London, working with general practitioners, demonstrated how the physi-cian's own feelings, attitudes, and behavior affected the outcome of the patient–doctor interaction and stated that the doctor's personality was his or her strongest therapeutic agent. Later, while psychiatrists were urging clinicians to ascertain the "story behind the story," anthropologists and sociologists showed how culture and society influenced patients' and physicians' thinking and behavior and pointed to the fact that Western microbiological scientific medicine was only one of many different concepts of illness and disease. George Engel in Rochester, New York, tried to combine these facets into a comprehensive biopsychosocial model of disease while Rolland, Doherty and Baird, and Medalie and Cole-Kelly developed models for the doctor–patient relationship. In the 1990s there has been a resurgence of interest in medical interviewing, and Bird and Cohen-Cole, followed by Lazare, Putnam, and Lipkin have classified the functions of good interviewing. In all of these, the quality of "listening to the patient" is often implied without being overly stressed despite its importance, as shown by Robert Smith, Stein and Appley, and some psychiatrists.

In this chapter, a number of stories and clinical anecdotes illustrate the effect of listening to the patient, which is not just an "active process" by the physician, but also implies that the physician has altered his or her way of thinking about the patient. In a sense, it is almost like changing from the biomedical outlook to something beyond it that includes an understanding of the patient as a person with his or her own beliefs and attitudes, necessitating an empathetic reaction and identification with the patient. These stories illustrate not only some remarkable patients, but also, I believe, remarkable physicians who went beyond their training to discover the core of the patient's story. To do this implies that the physicians themselves had achieved sufficient insight and understanding of themselves, often with the help of their patients or a clinical incident, so they were able to change their own thinking and attitudes and thus help their patients.

Each story in this chapter illustrates how the physicians learned sufficiently from their patients to change or modify their own attitudes and behavior with a resulting improvement in medical care and a heightened satisfaction and self-understanding for the physician. These stories from different geographical places with patients of varied beliefs show us that listening to and learning from patients is a universal attribute (with local variations) of primary care physicians. *Active empathic listening; seeing the patient in context; reflective and reflexive practice*—these are all keys to learning from patients. The results can be startling. In Dr. Miller's story, the physician learned to restore a soul, while in other narratives, the doctor found his or her own soul. In some of the stories in this chapter, the physician-writers received lessons in how to be small and humbled by the arrival of new life or how to accept needy help from a previously assisted patient. Sometimes it behooves the patient (like Melanie in Dr. Griffiths's story) to wait for the physician to learn to listen to her. Sometimes a patient (like Sonya in Dr. Phillips's account) plays the game of cat and mouse with the physician until he learns.

All physicians listen to the patient in one way or another; just a few (like those who wrote the stories in this chapter) not only listen, but also hear and learn. The motto "There is always another patient waiting to teach me some-thing new" may be a cure to many of the blues of our profession and our own personal dilemmas and anxieties. Acquiring the skills to do this may allow the doctor–patient therapeutic relationship to reach a deeper level of understand-ing with better outcomes for both the patient and the physician.

Melanie: The Path to Admiration

Frances Griffiths
Stockton-on-Tees, United Kingdom

I was new to general practice when Melanie started coming to see me. She was in her twenties, hugely obese, with scratched spots on her face and trunk. She dragged herself along while pushing her young child in her stroller. Her child, constantly pacified with candy, was very sticky from the sweets. When she came in the room an odor of sweat and chips exuded from her. She sat and moaned to me about her aches and pains and general malaise. My heart would sink when I saw her.

Nothing would have stirred me to go near her or listen to her if that hadn't been my job. I would have carefully avoided sitting next to her on a bus, in church, or at a community social event. I may have gossiped about her and used her as an example of "what the world is coming to." But I was her doctor and I had to let her come and see me despite these feelings.

At first I tried to find a cause for her pain and malaise and tried to sort her out. I did blood tests; I gave her prescriptions for her skin. I talked with the health adviser (a public health nurse) about her. I felt I was getting nowhere. She wasn't responding to my efforts, but she continued to come and see me. In my despair, I began to just sit still when she came to see me and let her talk, hoping she would then go away. I couldn't see any other way to cope with my sinking feeling. From the depths of my feeling of despair about Melanie, I began to hear her story. I also was stirred to read her story, the parts buried within her thick medical records.

She had a poor but stable upbringing, crossing swords with her father many times. She still saw her mum and dad, although they disapproved of most everything she did. She became pregnant at eighteen, married the baby's father, and moved with him into the council housing estate, public rental housing. It was an area infamous for its poverty, vandalism, thuggery, and more serious crime. While she was carrying the baby, her husband had a severe asthma attack and died. A few months later, she gave birth to a stillborn child. Melanie became depressed and was in and out of a psychiatric hospital, taking overdoses and slashing her wrists. She then became pregnant by another man, a man already married with his own children, who wasn't going to leave his family. She carried on with the pregnancy, needing treatment with insulin injections to control diabetes of pregnancy. Her second child was healthy, but she was now alone with a baby on the same difficult housing estate.

As Melanie kept coming to me and talking I began to notice that although the child was sticky with chewy sweets she seemed alert and happy.

She was growing and developing normally. Melanie began to look happier, she lost some weight, and her skin began to heal as she stopped scratching.

I began to admire Melanie. She had coped with more as a teenager than many do in a lifetime. To see her begin to put her life together was a privilege but still mixed with some anxiety when she came to see me. She was beginning to become happier and had a more positive view on life when further misfortune plagued her. Her mother developed breast cancer, and Melanie became so worried for her she started scratching again. Concurrently, the council started demolishing part of the estate where she lived. Her house was relatively new and was not planned for demolition. However, for three to four months there were fires started in the empty houses around her and bricks thrown through her windows. Melanie scratched her skin and visited me frequently. She managed to cope, and did so in a far better manner than I feel I would have in that situation.

One day Melanie came to see me, and we discovered she was pregnant again. Initially, my heart sank, but it was what she wanted and her boyfriend wanted to stay with her this time. Melanie managed to move to another area, and she did not come to see me anymore. I heard through her midwife that she went on to have a healthy child and had settled in her new home.

Although I found her difficult, part of me came to care about Melanie. I wanted to hear the outcome of her pregnancy after she left. I wanted to send a card to congratulate her, but I didn't. Part of me feared she might come back. I knew I still would not want to sit next to her on a bus.

I sometimes wonder why so much should befall one person. Further, how does one who appears to be without the strength or resources to manage cope better than one who does? Melanie did have an inner strength that gave her the ability to survive it all. She never stopped caring for her child, parents, or boyfriend despite all of her difficulties. What I took away from her experience was that she was the one who waited for me to learn to listen to her.

Passing: The "Norm" and Quality of Life

Mindy Smith
Chelsea, Michigan

Watching her walk into the office was painful. Her body would shift almost violently from side to side as she swung first one and then the other leg forward, leaning heavily on two canes. We had nearly exhausted the list of anti-spasmodic medications in an attempt to lessen the scissoring gait. The medications that worked best were so sedating that she could hardly keep her head up. Still we tried to find the combination that would allow her to function in her job and yet enable her to move from her desk to the files or walk down to the lunchroom with her co-workers.

She did find brief respite from the constant back pain (a result, I am convinced, of that jarring gait) by performing a series of exercises. Her job, however, left her so weary by the end of the day that eating, bathing, and bed were all that she could manage; so exercise was relegated to weekends. A chiropractor gave her a few pain-free moments as well. Her income, however, could little support the frequency of visits required to restore some semblance of alignment to her back before the intense spasms would pull her small bones in a thousand different directions. I contributed little beyond a handful of medications and occasional physical therapy to maintain the status quo; although I offered an ear, she rarely complained.

One afternoon she came to see me with a picture given to her by a friend who was a physical therapist. It displayed a high-tech wheelchair, the sort that racers use, capable of tight turns and requiring little effort to propel. "So what do you think?" she asked quietly. I looked at her face full of hope that I would understand her need to relinquish those canes. "It's a great idea," I said. "I can't believe we didn't think of this before. What's the point of expending all that physical energy at work when it makes your life so much harder?" I wrote out a prescription that day but secretly worried about whether her muscles would, in fact, weaken with this change.

The difference that the wheelchair made in her life was astounding. She eased herself through her workday, enjoying her freedom of movement and newfound speed. She found time and energy to complete her exercises daily and her pain was managed with less medication. I realized what a terrible disservice I had done, encouraging her to strive to be like "the rest of us," the able-bodied, upright folk who waste no time considering whether to make the Herculean effort to go down the hall to the bathroom or wait a bit longer to minimize the number of trips over the day.

Since becoming disabled myself, the lesson I learned through this young woman's struggle rings even more true. I strive to find simple yet creative ways to accomplish tasks, preserving strength and releasing those norms that no longer, or perhaps never, fit my needs.

Appearances

William R. Phillips
Seattle, Washington

Tanya was a twelve-year-old pregnant girl, a dropout and a runaway. She lived and worked on the streets. Despite cocaine use and secondary syphilis infection, her prenatal course was uncomplicated. Her labor and delivery went well, although neither her family nor her thirty-two-year-old boyfriend was there for support. When I discharged her from the hospital on the third postpartum day, I was concerned about her ability to cope with and care for her newborn son. I asked her to come to the office in a week, earlier than usual because I was worried about this high-risk mom and her higher-risk baby.

One week later she returned with her happy, healthy, well-dressed, and, to all appearances, well-cared-for baby. My concern continued despite the reassuring appearances. As always, I asked, "Any questions or problems?" "No," she assured me. I asked several more times during the well-baby examination, "Any concerns? Any worries? Anything you'd like to ask me?" She repeatedly assured me that she had no questions at all about caring for her new baby. I was still worried. Perhaps she did not know enough or was too embarrassed to ask any questions. How could this young woman—this girl, really—feel so confident and comfortable with the challenge of her first baby? How, indeed, when mothers with so much more education, prenatal preparation, family support, and resources had so many questions and so much insecurity?

I asked her a few questions to explore the limits of her knowledge. "What are you doing to take care of the baby's cord? How do you know when he has had enough to eat? What works best when your baby cries?" She had all the answers, it seemed.

My lingering doubts prompted me to confront her with one last question: "How come you know so much about babies?"

"Are you kidding?" she replied. "I have six older sisters. Every one of them has kids. Who do you suppose took care of all those little babies? My mother and me, that's who."

I realized that this twelve-year-old, despite all of her social and medical risk factors, did, indeed, have more experience caring for babies than did any of my patients with prenatal classes, professional careers, and PhDs. In assessing her risk factors and her appearance, I had stereotyped her without realizing the strengths that came from surviving the difficult life she had led so far.

"Olga": A Quadriplegic and Living Alone

Thomas M. Mettee
Chesterland, Ohio

Olga was born in Brussels on February 26, 1936, as the only child of Russian parents who escaped the Bolshevik revolution and famine. Her maternal heritage originated from St. Petersburg: her grandmother was a physician and a "Sunday painter"; her uncle followed in his mother's footsteps and was an artist and physician as well. Her own mother was a "beautiful, talented, intelligent, and courageous woman, liberated ahead of her time." Her paternal heritage originated from Ukraine and White Russia: her grandfather as a tsarist general with a bad temper and her father a tsarist military officer, "proud, brave, and stern." These inherited traits would secure her survival in very challenging future circumstances.

In 1951, when she was fifteen, her family immigrated to the United States, where she lived and attended art school in New York City. She married at age twenty and spent the next decade traveling, painting, and managing a textile design firm.

At thirty Olga gave birth to her only child and moved to Cleveland, Ohio. At this time she developed the symptoms of exhaustion, numbness, bladder incontinence, and a progressive loss of vision. These proved to be the first symptoms of multiple sclerosis, a diagnosis confirmed at the Cleveland Clinic when she was thirty-two. However, she became convinced that allergic and chemical exposures were the cause of her illness. Thus she designed and built an easy-care, low-chemical and low-allergy home on a concrete slab with drains on a seventeen-acre lot in rural Geauga County, thirty miles east of Cleveland.

Over the ensuing decade, she became progressively disabled through loss of leg power and required a walker and eventually a wheelchair. During this time she experienced marital difficulties and became dependent on her teen-aged son as her primary caregiver. By the age of forty-one Olga required a lift for making transfers to and from her bed. By the age of fifty she had become a blind, quadriplegic, total care patient depending on a patchwork quilt of caretakers: home health care agencies, local physicians, and friends. By this time both her husband and son had abandoned her. She was living alone with her only connections to the outside world a blow tube to her telephone and a lever system operated by her chin and tongue allowing her to control a pictureless TV set. Caregivers provided a bowl of liquid nutrition with a straw accessible when she turned her head to the right. At one point the health care community became so concerned about her safety that a referral was made to

Adult Protective Services. Outraged, she fired all professional caregivers and survived on the support of neighbors and friends.

Twenty-eight months before Olga died at home, I became her personal physician. This occurred through the emergency room on-call roster, which provides a physician for patients requiring hospitalization who do not have a physician on the staff. A rescue squad had been called to her home by a neighbor and she appeared in the emergency room as an emaciated, blind (with dense cataracts), quadriplegic (neurogenic bowel and bladder) suffering from severe, large bedsores over her lower back. She had a chronic urinary tract infection due to an indwelling Foley catheter complicated by bladder stones and a large stone in the right kidney associated with an abscess. Her protein malnutrition was severe. Her weight had dropped from 105 to 65 pounds with dangerously low levels of protein. She also suffered from an iron deficiency anemia.

After a month in the hospital during which time she received three transfusions, intravenous fluids, feeding tube nutrition, iron therapy, and care for her bedsores, she was ready to leave the hospital with her hemoglobin and body proteins near normal limits. She was adamant about being in her own home rather than a nursing home. She was prepared to die there without any further hospitalizations, partially due to the difficulty she experienced accepting traditional medical treatments. I agreed to do this if I could work with a local home health care agency with whom I had an excellent relationship.

The home health care service agreed to provide nurses and nurses aides only if they could be legally protected, since they were unable to provide the necessary twenty-four-hour care. As well, Olga had a prior history of "firing" the caregivers provided to her. I promised to make home visits at least once a month or more often when necessary. Thus we forged a care plan with the patient in the driver's seat. We rented an air bed that enabled her to lie on her back and reach fluids, her telephone, and her TV set. Aides arrived at her home at 7 A.M. and left at 5 P.M. A nurse visited daily. The rest of her time was spent alone. She refused all conventional drugs but accepted natural products and homeopathic remedies. Bowel control was managed with Metamucil and mineral oil followed by digital evacuation and occasional soap suds enemas. Her bedsores, which had only begun to heal in the hospital, were treated with wet-to-dry saline dressings, elastin cream, vitamin E oil, Kenalog spray, and even honey and Bag Balm. None of these was successful.

She introduced a garlic, thyme, and olive oil tonic, which was applied directly to her bedsores, and she drank a small quantity every day. The wounds healed. She used red hot cayenne pepper sauce as a pest control agent for ants, which would attempt to find their way to her sweet nutritious drinks in the bowl next to her head or crawl across her body. She introduced us to a yellow dock root (*Rumex crispus*)—a plant root rich in iron, vitamin A, vitamin C, and oxalic acid. It had long-term use in both Chinese and American Indian culture and was used in this country by pioneer physicians to "purify blood and treat skin disease." Her hemoglobin rose from 11 to 12 and her hematocrit rose from 33 to 37—both within normal range—after a five-month failure of iron supplements (ferrous sulfate) to do the same thing.[1]

Olga gained weight while her kidney abscess atrophied from the size of a softball to the size of a golfball without the use of antibiotics. She became healthy enough to engage the services of divorce lawyers and the court to legally secure her ability to stay in her own home until the very end. Her death occurred during her sleep on July 15, 1995, nine years after she was originally bedbound.

Epilogue

Olga taught me the power of listening to patients, accepting (when possible) their point of view and belief system, and working with them to achieve a comfortable resolution in a case of desperate physical disability. She was able to direct her own care with dignity and control the social and physical environment around her. With the support of a health care team created from friends, aides, nurses, social workers, physicians, lawyers, and community financial resources, she was able to knit together her once raveled sleeve of care.

1. Hemoglobin is the iron-based molecule in red blood cells that transports oxygen; hematocrit is the percentage of the volume of a blood sample which is occupied by red blood cells.

The Alternative Cancer Patient

Stanley G. Smith
Saskatoon, Saskatchewan

I recognized him immediately when he was shown into my office. I recalled that he was a freelance science writer who had interviewed me about a year earlier regarding the management of hypothermia. I even remembered his name—Harley Stevens.

"What can I do for you, Harley?" I asked, wondering if this was another interview he was soliciting, and glancing at my watch as I knew I had a full list of patients scheduled.

"I think I'd like you to be my doctor," he said, "so I set up an appointment to discuss this with you, as I do have some conditions before I make up my mind."

"Tell me what they are, and I'll tell you if they are acceptable to me," I said, reflecting on some of the bizarre requests that had been made of me in the past.

"Well, I refuse to be burnt, cut, or poisoned," he said.

I looked at this tall, thin, balding man, with a fuzzy ring of graying hair around his bald spot. His intelligent blue eyes held mine as though everything he had said was self-explanatory, and all he needed was my agreement. "Exactly what do you mean by that?" I asked.

"Well, I had cancer of the bowel about five years ago, and had it removed surgically. When I was attending for a follow-up examination about a year later, the doctor said he thought my liver was enlarged and they did an ultrasound, which they told me showed secondary spread to my liver. Now, I have a science background and I fully understood the implications of that, so when they offered me chemotherapy, I decided there and then that I would reject the triad of further surgery, radiotherapy, or chemotherapy—cutting, burning, or poisoning." He smiled and added, "That is why I left my previous doctor, who found my attitude unacceptable, and that is why I am coming to you with these provisions."

I have always found it hard to understand why some physicians have difficulty in accepting that patients may make different treatment decisions than those recommended by the physician. They seem to regard this as some sort of personal affront. Most of the time it is not, and physicians and other health care workers must learn to respect patients decisions in these situations. So I didn't find it particularly difficult to accept Harley's stipulations.

"I have no problem in accepting that you have the right to decide what treatment you will or will not consent to; every patient has that right. The converse of this agreement is that you accept that I am going to give you the best medical advice I am capable of. I will try to make sure that you understand the benefits and the complications of such therapy, and the consequences of not taking the treatment. If after that you decide you don't want the treatment, then I will have no difficulty in respecting your decision. I also intend to contact the cancer clinic and obtain a copy of their findings and impressions."

"That's fine with me, Dr. Smith," he said, extending his hand. I took it, we shook hands, and thus began a long alliance which goes on to this day.

"Let me tell you why I am here today," he said. "I have had diarrhea now for about two weeks and that's how my original tumor manifested itself. So I really want to know what's going on."

"Yet you're not going to accept any therapy, whatever the results of the testing?"

"Well, I didn't exactly say that," he said. "It depends on what you have to recommend. I also have some views and treatments of my own, that helped me get through the previous bout with cancer." My curiosity, of course, was piqued. Wondering what sort of a challenge I was taking on here, I asked, "What sort of treatments are you talking about?" He smiled patiently at me as if to say: I know you think I'm crazy, but I've got you interested anyway!

"I did a number of things when the doctors told me they thought the tumor had spread to the liver and that even with the therapies that they had to offer, my survival was strictly limited with no indication of a worthwhile quality of life. I decided that the prognosis I was being offered was so gloomy, that I was going to take my care into my own hands." Harley smiled again, "In other words, I decided that my health was too important to be left in the hands of doctors. I decided to do two things immediately. I decided to try some alternative therapy. Now, I am not a naive man, and I do have a considerable background in science, as I have already told you. Nevertheless, I decided to give laetrile[2] a try. I did not think it was a miracle drug, but if you have nothing to lose except a little money, even the remote possibility that it will do some good is better than nothing. You doctors don't seem to understand that. You are so busy protecting yourselves and so preoccupied with particular types of studies, that you forget that most of the great scientific and medical discoveries were serendipitous events. Alexander Fleming didn't need any studies to show that penicillin works. Anyway, I went down to Mexico and had a course of laetrile. How much a part that played in my survival, if any, I really don't know. But I am still here, so I don't discard the possibility that it helped. If I had another episode, I would try it again.

2. Laetrile, a drug made from apricot pits, is claimed by proponents to have antitumor properties. These claims have not been proved, and the drug is not licensed by the U.S. Food and Drug Administration.

"The other thing I decided was to remove all the sources of stress from my life that I possibly could, and this was the really difficult part of my regimen. You see to do that, I had to give up my job, my home, and eventually the woman I lived with. I had a regular, dull writing job, that didn't interest me very much. I gave that up in favor of freelance writing, which was something I wanted to do, despite the uncertainty of making a steady living at it. My mortgage was demanding so I got rid of that too. I sold the house, paid off the mortgage, and had about enough money left over to go down to Mexico for my laetrile treatment."

He paused here, and I thought this a good opportunity to bring the presenting complaint back into focus. As fascinating as this was, the waiting room was filling up with impatient patients.

In addition to this history, Harley had had diabetes for years and was on regular doses of insulin. Recently he had an infected foot, and had been on antibiotics for this for two weeks about a month earlier. It was following this that the diarrhea had started and persisted. I told Harley that his diarrhea might well be due to the antibiotics and to eat some yogurt to help replace his gastrointestinal flora. In view of his past history we did investigate his gastrointestinal tract, which was normal.

In due course I obtained Harley's test results from the cancer clinic. There was no doubt that he had a pathologically proven carcinoma of his large bowel, which was resected, and that subsequently he was found to have an enlarged liver, which when investigated by ultrasound was reported to be suspicious for metastases, but which the patient refused to have biopsied. At that point the cancer clinic lost track of him as he refused to come back for further follow-up after refusing any other treatment options.

Harley continues to visit me intermittently, usually to address some issue that is presenting as an immediate problem to him. I am concerned that he does not take his diabetes very seriously, and although he takes some insulin daily, he frequently changes the dose "because he knows how he feels." Sometimes he follows my advice, sometimes he doesn't. He knows all about the complications of diabetes, but he really doesn't worry too much about the tightness of control because from his interpretation of the literature, it really doesn't make that much difference. When I tell him there is evidence to the contrary now, he agrees to review the literature when he has time and will get back to me. He was hired as a public relations man for a major youth group, and he is currently very busy organizing the group.

The last time I saw him was some months before my absence from the department for a year's sabbatical. He wanted to talk to me about an interview he had with a noted veterinary researcher, who was researching a new substance that helps diabetics. It hasn't been used on humans yet, and he thought he would like to be the first, so he wondered if I might supervise his progress should he get the substance. Even when I told him I couldn't prescribe such a thing or be a party to using it, he was not deterred. He said he would take it himself, without my prescribing it and instead come in for his follow-up checkups more regularly. I have no doubt that when I get back to my practice after my sabbatical, Harley will be waiting for me with some new therapeutic regimen he has researched, devised, and would like to implement. We will just have to negotiate, and sometimes he will follow my advice and sometimes it will be so important, he will just have to take his care into his own hands.

Restoring the Soul

William L. Miller

Harrisburg, Pennsylvania

It is an ordinary night on call—maybe better than ordinary in this central Pennsylvania hospital since there had been no disasters and I was getting some sleep. I was nearly finished with internship and feeling more comfortable with managing the routines of sickness and calming the waters of acute emergencies. The terror and memories of long hours were already fading, replaced by confidence and the rush of a newfound sense of control.

The phone rings; I awaken with a start. Soon I am at the bedside of a young woman from Mexico with the signs and symptoms of shock. She speaks no English and looks pale as a ghost. Her chart notes a successful removal of her gallbladder two days earlier with an uneventful recovery. But now her pulse is thready and racing, her blood pressure falling, her eyes empty, her lips graying, her abdomen silent. Intravenous fluids aren't helping. Her arterial blood gases, complete blood count, electrocardiogram, and portable X-rays of abdomen and chest are normal. But her condition rapidly worsens. My calm is shaken; I am scared.

I sit beside her pale form and again put my sweating hand on her wrist, feeling the disappearing pulse as I search those lost eyes for help. Then I hear it, or think I do, or is it the eyes speaking? "Se pierde, se pierde" ("It's lost, it's lost"). The whispers awaken memories from my days as an anthropology graduate student working in Central America. "¡Susto!" ("soul loss") I uncontrollably blurt out. Her eyes fix on mine as if saying "Sí." I reach for the X-ray of her abdomen and hold it in front of her eyes pointing to the cloudlike images of gas and stool. "Your soul. It's here; it's back inside you." And I lay the X-ray over her incision. Her eyes widen and she clutches the X-ray to her body. Over the next hour her vital signs return to normal, her attending physician finally shows up and leaves, and she is able to tell me what happened.

She had been terrified of the surgery. That very evening, at her first look at the incision, she immediately became convinced that her soul had escaped through the incision during surgery. Death was imminent. She was relieved to see her soul still there. I never told her the radiologist's interpretation.

I kneel and kiss her hand in gratitude. She gently turns her head and smiles graciously. There are no more ordinary X-rays and no ordinary nights.

References

Ackerman, W. W. 1959. *The Psychodynamics of Family Life*. New York: Basic Books.
Anon. 1994. The ethics of learning from patients. *Lancet 344(8915): 71–72. (editorial)*

Balint, M. 1957. *The Doctor, the Patient and the Illness.* New York: International Universities Press.

Dubb, A. 1983. Learning from patients. *South African Medical Journal* 64:885.

Engel, G. L. 1997. The need for a new medical model: a challenge for biomedicine. *Science* 196:129–36.

Hirshberg, C., and M. I. Barasek. 1995. *Remarkable Recovery.* New York: Riverhead Books.

Kleinman, A. 1979. *Patients and Healers in the Context of Culture.* Berkeley: University of California Press.

Lipkin, M. J., S. M. Putnam, and A. Lazare (eds.). 1995. *The Medical Interview.* New York: Springer-Verlag.

Melnikoff, P. 1989. *Plots and Players.* New York: Bedrick-Blackie.

Rolland, J. S. 1994. *Families, Illness and Disability.* New York: Basic Books.

Salter, H. R. 1996. Learning from patients: unfashionable but effective. *Postgraduate Medical Journal* 72:385.

Smith, R. C. 1996. *The Patient's Story.* Boston: Little Brown.

Stewart, M. A., I. R. McWhinney, and C. W. Buck. 1979. The doctor–patient relationship and its effect upon outcome. *Journal of the Royal College of General Practitioners* 29:77–81.

Wheeler, H. B. 1990. Shattuck lecture: healing and heroism. *New England Journal of Medicine* 322(21):1540–48.

Family and Community

Reflections

Howard Brody

In the introduction to this book, Jeffrey Borkan makes the important point that *every encounter between doctor and patient is a cross-cultural event.* This becomes obvious to us when the physician is a Westerner treating a non-Western patient, but it is not obvious at all when the physician is a lifelong neighbor of the patient. Understanding why this observation is true for all encounters, and not only for "exotic" ones, is necessary for success in primary care, as the stories in this chapter attest.

What makes a medical encounter a confrontation between two cultures? At an easy-to-recognize level, this occurs because medical training is itself a process of acculturation into a world different from that of the laity. Among the critical features of the exceedingly complex medical culture is a need to see the world as a composite of problems with solutions, where the "right" solution is often independent of which person has the problem. Eric Cassell (1976) commented that when Hippocrates laid the groundwork for Western medicine by claiming that no disease was supernatural—that all diseases could be understood by the study of natural biological phenomena—he also laid the foundation for a medical practice in which *the physician no longer feels the need to speak to the patient.*

Success in medicine means solving or eliminating the problem, and not necessarily living a life that is satisfying and meaningful. This has led sociologist Arthur Frank (1995) to conclude that at least some patients—those with chronic illnesses, which by definition resist any final "solution"—will need to form themselves into self-sufficient communities of storytellers and witnesses, since physicians will be largely unable to hear or to tell the sorts of stories that are most important for the healing of these sufferers. Even those who reject this pessimistic interpretation of Frank, arguing instead that the well-trained primary care physician can and should enter into the patient's illness episode, admit that this will require an often intricate negotiation between the medical worldview and the patient's life experience and that the traditional ways of training physicians often neglect the skills needed for this negotiation (Levenstein et al. 1986).

At a deeper level, which is harder to discern, every medical encounter is cross-cultural because of our common humanity, and not merely because of some aspect of professional training. To be human is to be shaped inevitably by one's culture, but to be shaped in a way which is simultaneously and constantly influenced by our family background and by our own individual personality. No two people are members of a culture in quite the same way; simply knowing a list of cultural beliefs and practices is insufficient to understand how any individual within that culture will behave or what he or she will value.

Families are important social units for many reasons, but for the purposes of this chapter, we may usefully view them as minicultures (Huygen 1978; Baird and Grant 1998). Cultures teach us sets of beliefs and practices which locate us in the world and lay out for us an array of possibilities and limitations for living our lives. The culture instructs us that these ways of living a life are good; these other ways are bad (but still understandable and meaningful within the culture); and yet other ways of living are inconceivable and meaningless. Within the array of possible lives that a culture presents to us, our family often expands or narrows the set of options. Sometimes our family upbringing teaches us that we are special, capable people and need not be so tightly bound by culturally imposed limits as our peers. In other instances, the "family script" acts as a restraint on the options of the individual, a cage with a wheel on which the hamster may run ceaselessly while going nowhere. Each episode of illness is played against a backdrop of some family dynamic; the history and emotional needs of the family and the dynamic of the illness episode will inevitably influence each other.

Since we desperately need our families for intimacy and emotional nurturance, spending a lifetime running around a hamster's wheel might be an acceptable fate, so long as the only alternative seems to be to sunder one's family bonds completely. In Igor Svab's story, we might wonder why Anton the undertaker repeats the same futile action year after year—bringing home a new belle from the spa, only to have his son run her out of the house. Why not move to a separate dwelling where he can cohabit with whomever he chooses? But we finally realize that at some level, it must be more important to the elder Anton to maintain the family line and the family business as an intact social unit. Indeed, we could even speculate that it is precisely the knowledge that his son will keep each liaison brief and noncommittal that allows the father to play role of the ladies' man at the spa each year.

If culture, then, affects every medical encounter (Helman 1990; Fernandez, South-Paul, and Matheny 1998), what is the nature of its impact? In a classic paper, Kleinman, Eisenberg, and Good (1978) suggested that there are some universal needs humans bring to a healing encounter. When we are sick, we want to know the name of the sickness, what has caused it, what can be done about it, and who can help. To a large extent our culture will determine what is to count as a meaningful or acceptable answer to these questions. Jack Medalie, in his story of a case of pseudo-pregnancy among a group of Yemenite Jews, was disturbed by his awareness that his scientifically "truthful" explanation of what had happened and what had caused it was completely unacceptable to his listeners; but he wisely intuited that left to their own devices, the Yemenite community would attach its own preferred meaning to these events—even if the result was a further rift with and distrust of the Western physicians.

The medical culture, with its focus on objectivity and precise measurement, easily relegates this role of culture in the medical encounter to the periphery. After all, so long as one makes an accurate diagnosis and prescribes the correct treatment, what does it matter whether the talk one has with the patient and the family (and the larger community) is culturally "meaningful"? Adler and Hammett (1973) argued that culture, meaningfulness, and therapeutic success actually are integrally bound together. They claim for medicine and culture generally what Jerome Frank (1973) suggested more narrowly for psychiatry—that the true healing power was to be found in what all psychotherapeutic approaches have in common, and not in each one's distinct features. Adler and Hammett sought the critical common elements among healing practices in all human cultures as a key to the question of why the encounter between physician and patient can be therapeutic, independent of the precise treatment administered. That is, they searched cultural anthropology for the basis of what is often called the placebo response—that component of healing which is attributable to the medical encounter itself and not to any specific content of that encounter (Houston 1938; Novack 1987).

Adler and Hammett found two elements common to all healing practices, across all cultures: they *provide a meaningful explanation* for the sickness and *express care and concern* for the sufferer on behalf of the wider community. To this formulation, Eric Cassell (1976) would add the importance of indicating the *possibility of mastery and control over the illness or its symptoms*. When the patient experiences all these elements in a healing encounter, as happened in Jack Medalie's experience in rural South Africa, dramatic results may occur even in the absence of "scientific" diagnosis and treatment. Dominique Huas, by contrast, found himself battling a self- or family-imposed *nocebo effect* (a negative placebo response) for the same reasons—his patient clung to an explanation which made imminent death a virtual certainty, and the "family script" seemed to preclude any possibility of care from others or of taking control over his own fate. Dr. Huas's willingness to listen to the patient's story (thus establishing a caring bond despite the patient's fatalism) and his gradual reinsertion into the script of acts of control were probably instrumental in restoring the patient to full function and breaking the imprisonment imposed by the script.

The model of the placebo response suggests to us that certain messages or utterances from the physician, as filtered through the patient's culture, might either promote or retard healing. And this healing potential of the message is to a large extent independent of the "truth" of the utterance in purely biomedical terms. Jack Medalie describes three cases, two in which he tells a biomedical "lie" and one in which he tells the truth. He suggests in his account that he was most effective as a healer in the two cases where the truth was altered to fit better with the cultural expectations and context. If truth is best defined as "what works" (as the American pragmatist philosophers would have it), then cultural meaning may be more important than biomedical facts when we are in the business of trying to heal. David Morris (1997) made this point in calling for a "biocultural model" of the placebo response:

Medicine as a cultural practice generates in doctors and patients a powerful set of connected beliefs that underlie any therapeutic encounter. The belief that doctors understand illness gives many patients an automatic expectation of relief such that the mere appearance of someone in a white coat—or other potent cultural image of medicine—can produce a placebo effect. In ways both subtle and diffuse, we learn to recognize the cultural signs that promise relief, from aspirin bottles to surgery. Further, most people recognize and consume medical care only within the larger context of a cultural situation in which some are designated patients and others healers. The placebo effect thus belongs to an encompassing cultural narrative in which humans project their own self-healing powers onto a doctor or shaman or priest, who triggers relief through certain arcane rituals and prescriptions. Despite the progress of modern biomedicine, it is a narrative that has not changed for thousands of years. (p. 196)

Dominique Huas, in his struggle against the nocebo effect of his patient's family script, experienced no conflict of loyalty—he had to choose to side with the patient, and life, or to side with death. Aya Biderman faced a more difficult choice. In one sense, the medical team (including the anthropologist-psychologist-consultant) intervened brilliantly, "curing" all of the patient's psychiatric symptoms largely without the use of medication. But in doing so, they effectively sided with the husband and the paternalistic culture against the patient's own hesitant struggle for reproductive choice and power. It would have taken considerable wisdom, perhaps superhuman wisdom, to discern a course of action in this case which did not take sides in a way that could lead to personal and family tragedy.

Dr. Biderman's story reveals, among other things, the fact that one bit of counsel *not* applicable to the primary care physician is to hold the patient's and the family's culture in the deepest respect and not to muck around with it. Like it or not, we are physicians. Whether our approach is narrowly biomedical-technological or broadly biopsychosocial and spiritual, we are still trained to see the world as being not quite right, demanding that we muck about with it—else why would the patient have sought us out? Robert Like's story gives us a creative example of a somewhat bold act of mucking about—a Jewish physician offering religious advice to a Catholic couple quarreling about sterilization.

An intriguing aspect of Dr. Like's story is that the wife apparently takes more comfort in his statement of a traditional Hebrew teaching than she did in the pronouncement of the "liberal" Catholic priest her husband had previously consulted. Why was this so? The answer seems rooted in a concept addressed by almost all the stories in this chapter—the importance of *relationship*. When the husband consulted the liberal priest who approved of his having a vasectomy, the wife had no chance of forming a personal relationship with that individual. Dr. Like, by contrast, met with the two of them and spoke with them long enough for the wife to feel that she had been heard and understood. He revealed enough about his own religious commitments to make the couple feel that he had opened up to them, a sign of mutual trust. Dr. Like's comment about the overriding importance of "peace in the house" did not appear out of the blue—it is not, after all, the case that Jews believe in family harmony while Catholics valorize conflict and strife within the household. Dr. Like did not simply pluck from his memory any handy Hebrew phrase; he chose one that gives voice to the deeper values that he sensed were implicit in the way that both husband and wife were confronting their differences of opinion. Because of all these things, Dr. Like could join with this Catholic couple by owning his own Jewishness, much better than he could have by borrowing any trappings of Catholicism.

It is instructive to contrast Dr. Like's relatedness to his couple with Jon Neher's apparent distance from the people he serves in rural Washington. He admires them for their "toughness," yet somehow these people, his fellow Americans, seem exotic to him. When a couple offers him a gift of warmth and gratitude for his healing efforts, Dr. Neher feels obliged to pull away, muttering "It's my job," as if to ward off any chance at a true relationship. The story is ambiguous about why this is so. Is it because this is simply a rotation lasting a few months in residency, discouraging the young doctor from putting down any roots (Christakis and Feudtner 1997)? Is it because of other unsatisfactory relationships happening in the doctor's life at the same time, hinted at in the letter from home? The lesson Dr. Neher speaks of in the end is of "strength" rather than "toughness," having seen vividly, at the operating table, how softness and delicacy can repose within the tough shell. But the narrative allows us to see this delicacy only in a patient who is unconscious and unable to relate. Dr. Neher seems to have learned his lesson across a gulf, which remains unbridged through the duration of his story.

These stories explain why a group of distinguished primary care educators recently urged *relationship-centered care* as the essential paradigm now missing from medical education and research in the West (Tresolini and P-FTF 1994). Perhaps, it is suggested, we could finally come to manage the education of future professionals properly if we could somehow put these nested relationships at the center of the experience of becoming a healer, and emphasizing that all else—scientific knowledge, clinical skills, and so on—is critical precisely to the extent that it serves and extends those relationships.

The centrality of relationship as a way of both knowing and healing in primary care brings us back once again to the importance of local knowledge. One forms relationships not with abstractions, but with specific people, families, and communities. We see in the stories in this chapter the physicians' dedication to forming and nurturing these nested relationships within the context of a concrete knowledge of the culture. The stories illustrate that even caring physicians dedicated to these relationships may fail, but physicians neglectful or dismissive of these relationships will almost certainly fail. A commitment to a deep understanding of family, community, and culture is a part of the "universal knowledge" of primary medical care. But what this commitment yields, in the real world of practice, is always local knowledge. In this way we see once again why concrete stories are so essential to comprehending good medical care.

Sleepless Nights

Jack H. Medalie
Waterkloof, South Africa and Atlit, Israel

Since graduating from medical school, I have practiced in Africa, the Middle East, North America, and two armies. This great diversity in geographic regions has encompassed people of many cultural, racial, ethnic, religious, and socioeconomic groups. They each possess their own values and beliefs quite different from those I had been brought up with or experienced during my scientific biomedical Western-oriented education. Though these dilemmas sometimes gave rise to dramatic solutions, they were also the source of many sleepless nights spent worrying and wondering.

Exorcising Evil Spirits

I was on a six-month stint at a small hospital in northwestern South Africa near the Botswana border. The hospital staff—a senior physician and I— were responsible for a twenty-five-bed joint medical-surgical ward (with an attached operating room), an acute infectious disease ward (diphtheria, measles, and whooping cough were rampant), a chronic tuberculosis ward, and a daily outpatient clinic of about thirty patients. It would have been impossible to cope without the assistance of many devoted African nurses, especially two male nurses (Reuben and Simon) who recorded the outpatient medical histories before the physicians arrived. They also acted as interpreters when my three languages (English, Afrikaans, and Sesuto) and/or cultural knowledge were insufficient.

One morning, on completing the ward round, I found Reuben waiting for me. He told me that in the preceding week, in an outlying area, two young male adults had "laid down and died" because they had been possessed by the "evil spirit," which the folk doctor's remedies could not rid them of. This story was relevant, because another young adult male with the same condition had been brought to the hospital by his family, to see if "Western" medicine would help him.

On examination, I found a muscular adult male in his twenties lying quite still on the bed. He responded slightly to pressure over his eyes, but otherwise he did not respond to the examination process, which revealed nothing that could account for his semicomatose condition. A complete blood count and sedimentation rate, two tests which show infection or inflammation, were done immediately and were both in the normal range. Being unfamiliar with this condition, I asked Reuben to inquire from some of the "elders" if there was any cure. The reply was that the only way to stop the patient from dying was to remove (or exorcise) the "evil spirit" from his body. Thinking about this, I remembered seeing the effect of intravenous calcium and told Reuben to tell him that he would receive an injection which would remove the evil spirit. He would know that it was leaving his body when he started sweating. Reuben put his mouth near one of the patient's ears and relayed the message to him. I did not see any reaction from the patient, but Reuben assured me that he had heard the message. Thereupon, I injected a vial of twenty cubic centimeters (20 cc) of calcium intravenously. This had to be done with great care, for injecting it rapidly would cause the patient to perspire, but too fast an injection could cause cardiac arrhythmia and even death. After about 10 cc the patient was sweating profusely with a pulse rate of about 140 beats a minute. (At this stage, my own pulse was probably in the same range.) I then slowed the injection until the vial was empty. To my absolute amazement, within fifteen minutes the young man was sitting up and talking. Despite my reservations, the patient left the hospital some hours later.

That evening the village drums beat loud and long as the people thanked their God and spirits for saving the young man. I too retired, thankful the rapid injection had not killed the patient. Despite the success of the treatment and my immediate rise in status with the nurses and the villagers, I did not repeat the treatment!

Telling Truths I

The second incident occurred in Israel. Between 1949 and 1951 approximately fifty thousand Yemenite Jews were transported by plane from Aden to Israel in the "Magic Carpet" operation. In Israel they were put into three temporary "camps" which had been British army barracks until May 1948. One of these camps was at Atlit, a town some twenty miles south of Haifa. Atlit was near five rural settlements which I served as family doctor. With the consent of the settlement of which I was a member (Moshav Habonim) and of the medical organization that employed me (The General Sick Fund of the Histadrut of Labor), I worked full-time in the Atlit camp for the first three months after the camp was established, and then part-time for a further six months.

The Yemenites were a very distinctive group, having lived in Yemen since the destruction of the second temple (about 100 B.C.E.), although some historians claim that they arrived in Yemen even earlier. The majority had lived in isolated small groups or villages, while others had inhabited the towns of Tzana and Aden. Whereas the villagers had maintained most of their original religious and cultural values and behavior, those living in Aden had received some formal secular education and had more contact with the dominant culture. Many Adenites had learned English or French at school, in addition to Arabic; the villagers spoke only Arabic. The Atlit camp's medical team consisted of three physicians (one from Germany, one from Poland, and me); a number of nurses, most of whom had immigrated from Europe in the preceding few years; and a few administrators, who were mainly born in Israel. The common language between the physicians themselves and the administrators was Hebrew; the nurse spoke Yiddish; the patients, Arabic. There were usually at least three languages spoken from the time the patient started to the end of the session when the nurse gave the treatment (Arabic–English–Hebrew–Yiddish)!

Medically, the Yemenites were small, malnourished, pleasant people, a little bewildered by the speed of their transformation with a host of serious illnesses: trachoma, tuberculosis, chronic malaria (spleens sometimes at or below the level of the umbilicus), tropical ulcers of their legs, and so on. Some cultural issues that had to be overcome at an early stage included a demand for pita rather than regular sliced bread with their meals (pita was provided); insistence on the physicians tasting all food in full view of the whole dining room before they would eat anything (we did this); and refusal to have their children sleep in beds or cots (solved by putting the mattresses on the floor).

I read as much as I could about their culture, but every day was a challenge. Usually the challenge proved stimulating, but learning about their beliefs and values from the patients and my interpreter sometimes was depressing. My attempts to integrate this knowledge with my Western medical beliefs and knowledge were at times extremely difficult despite my best intentions.

A few months after I had begun working at the camp, I received an obviously pregnant woman about forty-five years of age, accompanied by a happy group of five or six middle-aged women who surrounded the woman as if she was something special. Through the interpreter I learned that the patient, who had been married for about thirty years, had never been pregnant before. In their culture, a married woman who did not have a baby (preferably a male) had not fulfilled her role as a wife and was held in low esteem. The woman's current pregnancy was regarded as a very good omen and everybody was happy. She had come that day because she was having contractions and thought she was in labor.

Encouraging a few of the women to stay in the room, I brought in a female nurse, had the interpreter stand behind a curtain (he could hear but not see us), and proceeded to examine the patient. Her abdomen was large but soft, but I could not feel the fundus of the uterus or any limbs of the fetus and neither could I hear the fetal heart. This made me uneasy, and after an animated discussion with all those present in the room, the patient reluctantly agreed to let me do a vaginal examination. This revealed a small nonpregnant uterus with no adnexal masses, and with a sickening feeling it dawned on me that the diagnosis was pseudocyesis (a false pregnancy). To give myself time to think, I called in my older physician colleague, who repeated the examination, agreed with the diagnosis, wished me luck, and quickly left the room. The interpreter, nurse, and I retreated to an adjoining room where we discussed our options. What if I told them that the baby had died? No, because then the family would want the body for burial. After discussing various options, I felt that I had no recourse than to tell them the "truth."

With the help of the interpreter, who was himself very uncomfortable in the role, I explained as best I could (based on a Western-oriented psychological interpretation) what I believed had caused her to believe she was pregnant and to go through the nine months of abdominal enlargement, even to having contractions, without a fetus being present.

The patient and her entourage were stunned by the news but gradually began to ask questions in a more aggressive and antagonistic manner. They eventually left the room after having made many derogatory remarks about me, the camp, and the country. They regrouped outside with the patient supported by others in the group—wailing, chanting, tearing their clothes, and casting sand at their heads as they left. The procession slowly disappeared, leaving behind a stunned interpreter, a frightened nurse, and a sad and confused physician.

I had told the patient "truth" as my Western-oriented education had taught me, but in so doing, I might have destroyed a woman and devastated her family and friends. My only hope was that they were able to rationalize or explain the false pregnancy in terms of their own cultural beliefs or explanatory models. Many subsequent nights were spent discussing and thinking how I might have done things differently. I still do not know the answer.

Telling Truths II

The third incident occurred in the late 1950s in Jerusalem when I was the medical director of the Family and Community Health Center in Kiryat Hayovel. One morning on arriving at work I saw two groups of people—one surrounding a young woman and the other a young man—waiting to enter the center. It transpired that the young woman and man had been married the previous day and, according to their religious custom, the bed sheet with bloodstains on it (from the rupture of the virginal hymen) had to be shown to representatives of the two families. Despite the fact that they had sexual intercourse, the sheet had no bloodstains on it. The families had then consulted with their rabbi, who suggested they go their doctor to determine if she had been a virgin on her wedding night.

If the physician determined that she was a virgin (the hymen had been penetrated but not torn), then the marriage would proceed and the two families would remain friends. If, however, the doctor declared that she had not been a virgin (an irregular, previously torn hymen), then the woman would be disgraced and the two families could be involved in a conflict. Historically, conflicts similar to this type had sometimes led to bloodshed and even murder to preserve the "family honor."

The young woman, who was very quiet during the whole process, was accompanied by her mother and mother-in-law. Following the interview, I brought in a nurse and asked the two older women to leave the room while I performed the examination. The hymen was irregular and had probably been torn sometime earlier, but when I looked at the young woman and saw the entreaty in her tearful eyes, I knew that this time I was going to "stretch the truth" a little. At the request of the rabbi, I wrote a note certifying that she had been a virgin at the time of the marriage. The relief in the young woman's demeanor and the joy of the young man and both families were adequate compensation for what I had done.

Happily, I can report that the young couple maintained a stable relationship and continued to use me as their family doctor for the next five years, during which time they gave birth to two healthy children.

A Religious and Ethical Dilemma

Robert C. Like

New Brunswick, New Jersey

In the course of a busy day, John, a thirty-four-year-old man, came to the Family Practice Center requesting information about a vasectomy. Since he had been generally quite healthy, I had not seen him often. I inquired about his reasons for desiring a vasectomy.

John came from a family where Huntington's chorea[1] had afflicted his grandfather, father, uncle, and older brother when they reached their mid to late thirties. Fortunately, he was, symptom-free but was chronically anxious about whether he would develop this hereditary, degenerative, neurological disease. John had been married for eight years. He and his wife, Diane, were devout Catholics. They had successfully used the "rhythm method" for contraception until two years earlier, when his wife developed irregular menses during a period of stress, and unexpectedly became pregnant. This triggered much marital turmoil due to uncertainty about whether the Huntington's chorea gene had been passed on to their unborn child. There were no pregnancy complications, and a healthy son was delivered. The marital difficulties continued, however, as both were worried about their child's future. There was a lot of arguing and tension between them, and they stopped having sexual relations due to their fear of another pregnancy.

John told me that he had become increasingly uncomfortable with this situation and had gone for advice "to a liberal priest who gave me permission to have a vasectomy. My wife, however, is adamantly opposed to this and consulted a more conservative priest who said that having a vasectomy is a sin and should not be done. I don't know what to do. I don't want my marriage to fall apart. It's not good for our son to see us fight. I also am so afraid of Huntington's chorea. Can you please help?" After an empathetic comment, I suggested that perhaps it would be useful for both John and his wife to come in together for a counseling visit. John readily agreed to this and thought that Diane would also agree. We scheduled a half-hour visit for the next week. So much for a simple office visit about the pros and cons of vasectomy.

During the week I had a chance to think and plan. How did both John and his wife really feel about the vasectomy? Were any other forms of contraception acceptable? How could they deal with the differing recommendations of the priests? Would speaking to a third priest break the tie? Perhaps the fact

---

1. Huntington's chorea is an inherited, chronic, progressive, degenerative disorder usually beginning between age thirty and fifty. It is characterized by irregular, spasmodic, involuntary movements of the face and extremities, and a slow, continual loss of mental capacity ending in dementia.

that two priests had given them different religious interpretations indicated that they were faced with a "free-will" decision. What about the possibility of genetic testing for Huntington's chorea? If John tested negative, the vasectomy question would become moot and both he and his son would no longer have the fear and uncertainty. On the other hand, if John tested positive, he would have the terrible knowledge of what his future would hold.

John, Diane, and I discussed these questions during their visit. Diane was very religious and dutifully observant; she was unalterably opposed to vasectomy and other forms of contraception. She was not interested in speaking to another priest. Neither felt comfortable with the option of genetic testing for Huntington's chorea; however, they both realized that their marriage was in trouble.

During the previous week I had thought about my role as a Jewish family physician and wondered how to reconcile my own personal beliefs and feelings about the situation. I decided to share with them that as a Jewish physician, I could not presume to tell them what to do. Nevertheless, I stated that from my own religious perspective, I felt that preserving *shalom bayit,* a Hebrew phrase for "peace in the house," was critical for both them and their son. The visit ended amicably. Both John and Diane said they felt better knowing that I was also religious and could understand their predicament.

A month passed and I subsequently received a letter from John, who informed me that he had undergone a vasectomy. Diane, initially very unhappy, felt better after John went to confession where the priest helped him atone for his sin. The stress in their marriage had lessened, and they were becoming sexually active again. He still was extremely worried about the Huntington's chorea but hoped for the best.

Family Curse: "The Psychosomatic and the Danger of Death"

Dominique Huas
Paris, France

In May 1984, a patient of mine, Mr. K, came to see me. He was then thirty-four years old, a technician, married and the father of a thirteen-year-old boy. I knew from his past history that Mr. K's father had died when he was a teenager, leaving him and two sisters without a father. He was a sportsman and enjoyed cycling and sailing. He did not speak much and appeared disheveled, but he still gave the impression of being a kind-hearted man.

He came to my office with a fever, complaining of pain in his right calf, which had had been bothering him for fifteen days. The diagnosis of phlebitis was easy to make and the remainder of the clinical exam was normal. Laboratory tests revealed no coagulation trouble, and there was neither a personal nor a family history of such problems. Mr. K insisted on being treated at home and vehemently refused hospitalization. I prescribed heparin injections, which quickly achieved the desired anticoagulation. His fever quickly disappeared and the pain diminished. However, two weeks later the edema still persisted. The right calf was four centimeters larger in circumference than the left. I informed him of my concern that he had phlebitis, an inflammation of the veins of his leg, and explained the need for hospitalization. His fear of hospitals was evident as he became pale upon the mention of admission. I did my best to calm his anxiety without attempting to understand its origin. After much discussion, he finally accepted the decision.

Thirty-six hours later, Mr. K experienced a severe pulmonary embolism,[2] which obstructed 85 percent of the blood vasculature of both his lungs. With treatment, the blood clots and the phlebitis resolved and his lung perfusion — the flow of blood through his lung tissue — recovered almost completely. Plans were made for another hospitalization within two weeks to finish the workup of the etiology of the problem, and he was begun on outpatient therapy to prevent further clots.

Resignation in the Face of Death

On July 18, Mrs. K, very worried, rang me to let me know about her husband's health. The day before his second hospitalization, he had felt pain in the calf. At the hospital, the diagnosis of recurrence of phlebitis with an exten-

---

2.   Pulmonary embolism is a blood clot to the lungs, usually coming from the veins of the pelvis or lower extremities.

sion to the inferior vena cava was made. In addition to that, Mr. K began to speak about his death.

When he was moved from the intensive care unit to a regular ward, I visited Mr. K and found him very depressed. After his first stay in the hospital he had felt reassured, but he did not understand the necessity of a second hospitalization, and this brought back his anxiety even stronger. Withdrawn into himself, he did not want to speak about his fear. My perplexity, the seriousness of the situation, and the vital risk I felt he was in required that I intervene. I explained my doubts to him concerning the etiology of the increased severity of his illness. There did not seem to be any acceptable rationale for his prediction of impending death. However, I concluded that his phlebitis and pulmonary embolism could not be coincidences. The illnesses were spreading from within his own determination of his death. To stop this pathological succession of signs and symptoms, which I found suicidal, I felt that it would be better managed if we could discuss the rationale behind his intense fear.

The Family Curse

In time he opened up: "To me, the hospital only means death! Moreover, I have always known I would die between thirty-five and forty." He told me privately that his time had come. He was almost resigned to die. His father died as a result of a working accident, his legs crushed (association with the calf pain?). His grandfather died as a result of tuberculosis of the lung, which he seemed to analogize to his pulmonary embolism. Therefore, the men of the family were to die between thirty-five and forty: this had always been in his mind and in the family unconscious. Mr. K's son was thirteen, coincidentally the same age Mr. K was when his father had died. With the admission of this anxiety deeply embedded in his subconscious for years, Mr. K burst into tears like a little boy. He foresaw his own son's destiny perpetuating the "family curse." We spoke that day for a long period of time and continued to discuss these issues in the days that followed.

After his hospitalization, he regularly came to my office. He scrupulously took his anticoagulant tablets daily. He was, however, eager to cease taking them despite the recommended lifetime of treatment. I told him it was impossible to think of stopping before the fateful start of his fortieth year. He understood that. In October, he went back to work on a part-time basis. The routine visits followed one another, without any evidence of further health problems.

The End of the Spell

In January 1985, varicose veins appeared on his right calf. In December 1986, an ocher dermatitis—a yellow skin discoloration and inflammation—appeared. The development of ulcerative skin changes from the varicose veins required surgical intervention, therefore a hospitalization. We calmly spoke about it and I told him there was no emergency. His fear of the hospital had become blurred, but the hospital continued to represent a death symbol. To cope with his need for surgery, he decided to circumvent the hospital and sought treatment at a private clinic.

This approach reassured me. He stated that he had rationalized his fears and was no longer convinced that he was near death. Mr. K was relaxed, for the "private clinic is not the hospital." I felt he was confident and in control of his situation, and I relayed this to him.

In February 1987, Mr. K underwent surgery for his varicose veins with no postoperative complications. Ten days later, we mutually agreed to stop the anticoagulant treatment since he appeared to be out of the high-risk category. Mr. K had been taking the medication three years. Since that day, I have not seen him, but I know he is well, alive, and forty.

Epilogue

In the story of Mr. K, the hospital and the medical model have been the dramatic source of the family curse. Did the power of the mind have a pathological role? The anxiety of a hospital admission certainly had an impact. In retrospect, would the avoidance of the first hospitalization have altered the posthospitalization trauma and the disease process? Probably not, but I did not pay enough attention to Mr. K's reluctance and fears.

Mr. K did not discuss his anxiety with me or the hospital doctors. His apprehension of discussing his feelings of impending death and his resignation to his fate only reinforce two beliefs. The first is the power of a belief in fate and our own mortality. The second is the power of the medical model. It is very easy for a patient to become passive in the treatment process and carry out the "sick role." I had to push through his reluctance to speak out and to accept treatment to end what he considered to be inevitable. He was able to tell his story only after suffering and fulfilling his contract—at least partially—in accordance with the "family unconscious."

I am convinced that it was my role as the physician to coax Mr. K to confront his fears for two reasons. The first is medical. After the second hospitalization came the definite possibility of a third admission. The submission to what he believed to be his fate and the lack of control Mr. K felt he had over his own treatment and course of his disease allowed the illness to continue to control his body. When he became able to choose the place and the date for treatment, he began to control his own destiny. After the successful surgery, the anticoagulant treatment could be stopped; this allowed him and his family to put a close to the painful series of events.

The second rationale was based on a humanistic model. Mr. K, through the control he gained over his own body and his role in his own treatment, was able to overcome what he believed was the family curse. He had opened his own future and perhaps modified his son's.

Did words, empowerment, and a kind ear stop the death process? Such a treatment method cannot be part of the medical model or be confirmed from scientific testing. There is no doubt, however, that utilizing good listening and speaking skills can enhance the patient–doctor relationship and play a therapeutic role. In this case, it saved a patient's life.

Last Day in Omak

Jon O. Neher
Renton, Washington

The wilderness still lurks in the back canyons and forests of the Okanogan Valley. Only a narrow strip of land along the river has been domesticated with apple orchards, wheat, and cattle. A few small towns dot the riverbanks. The people of these towns are still people of the frontier. A mystique of strength, self-reliance, and just plain ruggedness permeates their lives. I was spending a few months in this remote rural Washington State community as part of my residency training in family medicine.

As I looked at the screw sticking out of the bottom of Jimmy's foot, I knew that injury and disease also lurked in the Okanogan's shadows. Jimmy, age three, had been running around in a pasture barefoot when he stepped on a forgotten construction screw. The X-rays showed it to be embedded about an inch, but luckily it had not struck bone. I tugged at the screw gently. Jimmy winced. The screw did not budge. I was going to have to unscrew it to get it out.

Jimmy looked at me with a huge pout on his lower lip. He wondered what I was going to do. I wondered what I was going to do. General anesthesia or a large dose of narcotics would be dangerous. Local infiltration of anesthetic would be painful. I sent the nurse to get a screwdriver. "Take it out," he said.

I sat on the examining table next to Jimmy. He was wearing a scaled-down version of the overalls most of the local farmers wore. "You know Jimmy," I said, "I am going to have to take the screw out of your foot. It's going to hurt, and there is nothing I can do about that." He frowned but nodded his head. "But I want you to be in control of how much it hurts. Can you count to five?"

"One, two, three, four, five," he muttered.

"That's good. Now as I take the screw out, I want you to tell me how much it hurts. One means it hurts a little, two means it hurts a little more. Three means that it hurts a lot. Four means it hurts a whole lot more, but not so much that you can't take it. Five means it hurts too much. If you say 'five,' I'll stop. Do you understand?" Again, a nod and a frown. Jimmy's mother sat by silently.

The nurse then returned with the screwdriver. "Here we go," I said gently. "Remember, if the pain gets to a 'five,' I'll stop." I inserted the screwdriver into the notch on the head of the screw and slowly, steadily started to turn.

"Three!" Jimmy yelled. "Threeee! . . . Four. . . . **Four.** . . . **Four!**" His voice was shrill and tears flowed from his eyes, yet he held his foot rock steady. His mother looked like she was in shock. I broke out in a cold sweat. I continued to turn the screw.

"If you want me to stop, say 'five,'" I said through clenched teeth. The screw was starting to loosen.

"**Four!**" he cried. "**Four, four, four, fou—**" The screw fell onto the table. Instantly his mother was up and had gathered him into her arms. Over her shoulder Jimmy stared at me fiercely. He rubbed his dirty wet cheeks with his fist.

"I didn't say five," he said.

"No, you didn't say five." I looked out the window for a moment to compose myself. A drop of sweat trickled down between my shoulder blades. I stared through the summer haze up the Okanogan River to the little town of Omak and wondered, how is it that even the children are strong?

Later in the afternoon, my nurse told me that I had an unscheduled patient—a pregnant woman who had come in because of cramps and bleeding. I opened the exam room door and saw a trail of blood that ran from the door to the examining table. There, a large woman in her mid-thirties lay, ready to be examined. I introduced myself. She told me her name.

"How far along are you?" I asked.

"Four months." Her voice was hard.

"When did you start bleeding."

"Yesterday."

"Have you passed anything other than blood?"

"A few clots is all."

"Okay. Let me take a look." I sat down at the end of the examining table. As her knees fell apart, a macerated fetus was exposed, half protruding from her vagina. It was gray and flat as a piece of cardboard. Obviously, it had died in the womb several weeks earlier and was only now being expelled. I swallowed loudly, glad that the woman could not see the color drain from my face. "Five," I said to myself. "Five, five, five!"

I called for the nurse. She was in the room immediately. She saw my face and put a hand on my shoulder. "I'll get a basin," she prompted.

"Um . . . uh, yes. Get a basin. And some ring forceps." With the forceps, I extracted the fetus, then placed it in the basin and covered it with a towel. "I'm afraid that you've lost the pregnancy," I said. "You'll need a D & C[3] to stop the bleeding, but you should feel a lot better in a couple of days."

"Do I get to see it?" she asked, not moving.

I looked at her face. There was no expression. I brought the basin over to

---

3. D & C, dilation and curettage, is a procedure to dilate the uterine cervix and remove the superficial lining of the uterus and uterine contents.

her and uncovered it. For a long moment, she looked down at the little gray half-moon that floated in a crimson sky. "Okay." The gesture she made with her head indicated that the basin should be taken away. "I just wondered what it looked like." She closed her eyes. Her lashes were wet but no tears flowed. "Bud and I will try again next year."

She spoke of the fetus as if it were a field of winter wheat mowed down by hail. I felt a little shaky. As the nurse began to prepare the room for D & C, I stepped outdoors for a moment. Across the river, afternoon thunderheads gathered in the arms of the mountains. There was a taste of moisture and electricity in the hot breeze. To my left, a field of cows took no notice of me or the thunderheads. They chewed on their cud. I chewed on an image of the woman's face as she gazed in the basin. Tough. Tougher than I had been, anyway.

Heavy cloud shadows drifted over Omak. There would be rain later. I turned and went back into the clinic. I thought that the rigors of medical training had hardened me. But I was certain that this small town on the edge of the river concealed stores of strength that I could not imagine.

The D & C took a long time because my hands were still shaking.

After my last clinic patient, I went over to the hospital's intensive care unit (ICU) to see Mr. Gunderson. I had admitted him about a week earlier with chest pain. The electrocardiogram (EKG) had revealed that he was having a massive heart attack. With therapy, his initial pain had been controlled and the attack was abated. But every two or three days since his admission, he had suffered a recurrence of his pain as more and more of his heart muscle died. After several such episodes, I was dejected. But no matter how much of his anatomical heart blackened within his chest, Mr. Gunderson's resolve never wavered. His wife of sixty-five years was his constant companion and, as I entered the ICU, she was in her usual chair by his bed. I interrupted a conversation about their garden. Seeing me, he looked up and said, "I'm ready to go home, Doc." It was a statement that he made at least twice a day. Today, the tone reminded me of Jimmy's stern, "Take it out."

"Well, you've gone a little over twenty-four hours without any more chest pain. If things stay quiet, I'll have you out of bed some tomorrow. I've got my fingers crossed for the middle of next week."

"Good." He smiled and looked over at his wife. "We can watch the fall colors come in." He had a lot of gumption, but he still looked very tired. His breathing was coming harder and his feet had started to swell. "And it's going to be time to start harvesting the garden soon."

"Is he going to be able to work outside when he goes home?" Mrs. Gunderson asked. "That's what he enjoys most." She did not look at me as she spoke, but only at him. There was a profound tenderness in her voice. It was not the fearful voice of someone facing widowhood.

"I don't think he is going to feel up to it right away," I said. In truth, I was not even certain that he would be going home. There was a long silence while they gazed at each other. I felt like an intruder in some sacred place.

Finally, Mr. Gunderson spoke. "Doc, Ruth and I have been married for as long as I or anybody else can remember. And each and every one of those years was wonderful. We both wanted you to know that we appreciate your efforts to keep us together as long as possible."

I could not think of a reply. His stubborn determination was not for life but for life *together*. Unable to share what I was feeling, I finally shrugged my shoulders and said, "It's my job."

As I left the hospital, the setting sun lit the underside of the thunderheads that marched down the Okanogan River valley and the fetal moon was blotted out by rolling black clouds. A stiff wind rattled the dry baby's breath that grew along the road. Most of the cows in the nearby field had moved under some cottonwoods. The leaves fluttered like mad, silver dancers.

I walked to my apartment a short distance away. There was a single letter for me in the mailbox. I took it out, unlocked the door, and went inside. The apartment was large but contained only a bed, a card table, and two folding chairs as furniture. I took a can of chili out of the cabinet and started to fix dinner. When the chili was hot, I sat down with it and opened the letter. It was from a woman I knew in the city. She said that she missed me. She hoped that I was working things out for myself. She said she hoped that I would be coming back soon. I set the letter down. Closing my eyes, I felt for a brief moment the painful desperation that lurked in my own shadows.

The phone rang at three in the morning. It was Dr. Jarvis, the only surgeon in the valley. "Get your buns over here, fishbait! I've got a hot appendix." He hung up. I stumbled out of bed and into some scrubs. As I walked out into the night, running water gurgled down the rainspouts and gutters. The black street glistened in the hospital's security lights. While I slept, the storm had come and gone.

I walked into the operating room, masked, and scrubbed. The nurse helped me into a sterile gown and a pair of gloves. Dr. Jarvis was already there, placing sterile drapes over an anesthetized female patient. Soon she was submerged in a sterile blue ocean—her abdomen a small tanned island of flesh in its midst. As Dr. Jarvis and I took our places on opposite sides of that island, he told me the story. Twenty-two years old with a history of pelvic inflammatory disease, she had presented with right lower quadrant pain. Fever, 102° F. Definitely peritonitis.[4]

Dr. Jarvis drew his knife across the skin, cutting a neat red line. Deftly he worked his way down through the abdominal muscles into the peritoneal cavity. In less than fifteen minutes, the diseased appendix was exposed. It was so hard from inflammatory infiltration that it stuck straight up out of the

---

4. Peritonitis is an inflammation of the lining of the abdomen.

wound. Seeing the decidedly phallic effect, Dr. Jarvis laughed. Wrinkles appeared around the eyes of the masked scrub nurse, betraying her hidden smile. We had all noticed the resemblance. Soon the appendix was out and in the pan. Dr. Jarvis placed his hand into the wound to search for other anomalies. I was sleepy and let my mind wander. Someone turned on the radio in the operating room. An old love song was playing and Dr. Jarvis joined with it. His voice was pretty bad but the melody was recognizable. I found myself thinking about love rather than tissue planes.

Dr. Jarvis pulled from the wound part of the uterus and the accompanying fallopian tube and ovary. They glistened under the operating room lights. Their arrangement on the drapes was strangely beautiful.

"You know, she said she was having trouble getting pregnant," Dr. Jarvis said casually. "I guess this is why." He held up the soft fimbriae, and there, delicate as the wing of a dragonfly, a band of tissue separated the opening of the tube from the ovary.

I thought of all the couples I had seen who wanted children and could not have them. Did they know the frailty of the obstruction—one gossamer layer? Dr. Jarvis split it with an overly dramatic swipe of his scissors. "There. Tell her that she will need to be careful now." I smiled, amused by the surgeon's flirtation with omnipotence. Still, I could not take my eyes off the organs laid out pink against blue. Delicate! I almost feared to touch them—how easily all might be torn. And I realized that this is where we all come from, and we are never really tougher than our fragile first home.

Dr. Jarvis was not so reverent. He wrestled all the parts back down into the abdomen and began to sew. I helped with tying and cutting sutures. To pass time, Dr. Jarvis started to sing along with the radio again—this time butchering the harmony. Another love song.

"I'll bet it's not like this back in the city, eh?" he bellowed, throwing a wink and a stitch my way.

"Nope!" I laughed and my thoughts drifted away again. Soon the patient would scar and the scar would be tough. But it was a toughness of shell only, a reaction to this harsh thing called life. The innermost parts would always be delicate.

A short while later, I stepped out of the hospital and decided that it was time to go home. I had learned important lessons of strength which I would carry with me forever.

The Undertaker

Igor Svab

Ljubljana, Slovenia

During my first week in practice, an elderly man came to my office complaining of general malaise and insomnia. He told me that his name was Anton, and he wanted my opinion as to whether he would benefit from a short stay at a spa. The eldest son in a large family, life had not been easy for him. He married quite late and his wife had passed away when their only son was eighteen. Rather than remarrying, Anton had decided to live with his son in the same house. Unfortunately, they did not get along well and quarrels between father and son were common.

He went on to relate that it was a family tradition to give the firstborn boy the same name; his father, son, and grandson were all Antons. He was a carpenter, and it was also a family tradition for the firstborn boy to take over the father's trade. His son had begun taking charge of the business, but it was still in his name. His grandson was also showing interest in the profession. The business was doing well and he could not complain about a lack of orders.

I took a medical history as part of the office visit. Anton had never been seriously ill, though lately he had developed problems with eyesight and shortness of breath during fast walks. He attributed his good health to hard work and to a habit of eating garlic—indeed, he smelled heavily of the evidence.

Overall, I found that he was remarkably fit for his eighty-five years of age. I recommended that he visit a spa and bid him good day.

The rest of his story was told to me by the nurse who was working with me and by the colleagues in the health center, who knew Anton quite well. They told me that the woodwork of my patient was of a peculiar kind. In fact, he was an undertaker.

Although being an undertaker was an honorable profession, it was not a very popular one. There are many myths of the trade, and undertakers seldom publicize their work. Anton's family had decided long ago to describe themselves as carpenters, although everyone in the community knew what their work was all about. Anton had successfully created a myth around himself. Rumors abounded about him. Due to his old age, people even started to wonder out loud whether he would ever die.

Anton had made it a practice to visit every new general practitioner. He felt that the doctor should know the undertaker and that they should respect each other, because they shared an important relationship to death.

His relationships with women were also somewhat strange. True, his wife had died early; nevertheless, he was not living the life of a monk. He had a habit of going to a spa every year to get away from his son and to get acquainted with older ladies who were visiting there. Quite often he arranged for one of them to come to the village for an extended visit. However, none stayed long.

The superstitious women in the town were convinced that he had an "evil eye." It was believed that if you came across him when he was in a bad temper and he looked at you in a certain way, you were doomed. Occasionally he would utilize the superstition to bring fear into others' lives. One day he got drunk in a local pub and looked at everyone angrily, stating: "You may do whatever you want, but one day you will all be mine."

The flow of his customers was secured and quite closely linked to the work of the general practitioner. Therefore, he and I came into contact quite often. He treated me with respect and, to my embarrassment, always saluted me on the street. He was especially attentive when I was returning from a home visit of an elderly or seriously ill patient. He was well informed of their health status and was not ashamed to ask me on the street for my prognosis.

His application for a spa was processed after a few weeks and he left shortly thereafter for his stay there. Upon his return, he visited me in the office saying that he felt much better. He had regained his strength and felt like a young man again. I soon discovered that the reason for this dramatic improvement was not the effect of the spa's treatments, but rather the influence of a widow he had met there. He had decided to bring her to live with him and had promised to marry her. She would inherit the trade. His son, however, ensured that the romance did not last long. Upon hearing the news of their plans of marriage, he took a plank and beat them both. The bride-to-be left in tears the following day and the romance was over. Anton did not come to my office, although after the beating he sustained, I felt certain that he would need me.

In fact, I never saw him again in my office after that incident. When I met him on the street, he looked like every other old man I have known. He was still saluting, but the sparkle in his eyes was gone. He stopped teasing women and going to the pub.

One night when I was on call, I received a phone call. The calm and familiar voice of Anton's son asked me to come, since his father was not feeling well. When I arrived, old Anton was lying in his bed, dead. He was already washed and fully dressed, with a rosary between his fingers and candles lit in the room. A luxurious coffin was already prepared in the basement.

During the next months his son took over his trade. He modernized the business: he bought a new car and employed a worker to do the digging, which he had been forced to do for many years. The women did not fear the evil eye of this undertaker. Some things did not change, however. The sign on the house was still the same, and the people were still saying: "Anton will take you sooner or later." However, they were now referring to another, younger Anton from the dynasty of Anton the undertakers.

An IUD with a Special Meaning

Aya Biderman

Beer-Sheva, Israel

She was a young Ethiopian mother of two young girls, one and three years old, who came to my office with her elderly mother. I knew her quite well. Her name was Simcha, meaning "joy" or "happiness." Her nonverbal communication conveyed quite the opposite message: she appeared very sad, quiet, and despondent. The older woman informed me that her daughter had not been eating. I gently asked the young mother about this in Hebrew, a language which she knew, but she would not respond. Instead, Simcha sat very quietly, her eyes looking down at the floor. Not giving up, I attempted to solicit the help of another Ethiopian immigrant as an interpreter; still, no clear answers were ascertained and she continued to stare at the floor. Her physical exam did not yield any further information. With some hesitation, I suggested that she return home with her mother and come back if the situation did not improve in a few days or if another problem arose.

Two days later she came back with her mother, appearing even more quiet and drawn. The worried mother said that her daughter still did not eat, would drink only a very small amount of tea, and did not do any of her regular tasks at home. She added that Simcha stayed in bed all day. I again attempted to talk with Simcha. She refused to answer. I requested that the mother leave so Simcha and I could speak alone. It took a long time to get her to open up and answer any of my questions, and even more time to get her to drink some tea. I had to hold the cup and feed the tea to her. I felt more and more uneasy. "What is going on?" I asked myself. It seemed rather obvious that Simcha was disturbed about something, but what was it?

I spoke with her husband and asked for an explanation. His responses were strange; something about having her IUD (intrauterine device) taken out, but he thought she might have had some illness. Still the picture was very unclear. At this point I decided to consult with a psychiatrist, and it took two more days to admit Simcha into the psychiatric hospital for investigations. She was now in a type of stupor referred to by the psychiatrists as "catatonic."

I was extremely puzzled. I could not understand what was wrong, but my gut feeling was that there was an Ethiopian cultural component to this woman's actions. I decided to consult with an anthropologist-psychologist friend, with whom I had studied a few months before, during a course about Ethiopians. The resulting phone consultation was very fruitful. First he said he knew what I was talking about. Simcha was experiencing, literally, the "eating cessation syndrome" of Ethiopian women. He had seen a few cases of this syndrome and also had written some articles about it, which he gave me. He was also willing to come to a meeting with the psychiatric team on the ward where Simcha was hospitalized.

It took some days to organize this meeting, but finally we did it. After juggling schedules, we brought together my anthropologist-psychologist friend and the ward staff, including two psychiatrists, the social worker, and one of the nurses. Meanwhile, the psychiatrists, who could not get Simcha to speak to them at all, had proceeded with a narcoanalysis. (This is a psychiatric assessment under partial anesthesia and helps in cases where there is a refusal to cooperate.) During narcoanalysis they were able to get Simcha to tell them the whole story. The psychologist-anthropologist did not want to hear about that, however. He went straight to the husband, shook his hand in the Ethiopian manner, and greeted him in the Ethiopian language. Then he went to talk with Simcha, who was still very quiet and withdrawn.

After about thirty minutes, he came back and told us what the psychiatrists knew from the narcoanalysis. The crisis started when Simcha, having two young girls, had decided to have an IUD inserted. She did not tell her husband about it, and the gynecologist did not ask whether her husband approved. In Israel, a woman does not need her husband's consent to have an IUD, but this is not the case in Ethiopian culture. Somehow Simcha's husband found out about the contraceptive device and became very upset. He demanded that Simcha take the IUD out. Frightened, she did what he asked. She was nonetheless very unhappy with the situation. At that point she decided to tell her family, and she met with her brother, who was the head of the family after her father died. In the Ethiopian tradition, the wife speaking with her family is a sign that she has serious problems with her husband. Her brother was willing to defend her, but she did not want a divorce from her husband. At that point, she was put between two very strong forces: her husband and her brother. She felt that she had no alternatives, which caused her to become "paralyzed," and she stopped eating as a means to commit suicide.

After the session, the anthropologist told us about the eating cessation syndrome, which is an Ethiopian reaction to being depressed and under pressure. We discussed the steps we needed to take in Simcha's therapy. During the following week, Simcha received psychotherapy on the ward with the social worker and made progress toward recovery, without any medications. She started eating and became more talkative. She was discharged soon after and returned home to her husband and family.

We sensed that the husband required some intervention as well. He was seen by a male social work student in the family practice unit, who helped him get back to his normal life after the crisis. The husband promised to look after Simcha and take good care of her. The couple was encouraged to go to an Ethiopian therapist who was the traditional healer for family problems. However, the couple refused, stating that they did not want to keep these traditions. We talked with Simcha's mother and brother about what had happened and they agreed to help Simcha return to full function. In the following months, we kept in close contact with this family to ensure that everything was back to normal.

About a year later the couple had another baby girl and within the following three years they had two more boys. The youngest is now three months old. I saw Simcha last week and asked her if she considered having a break after this baby. Slowly and quietly she said, "My husband, he doesn't want me to have anything. . . ." I felt deflated; I felt I had failed her. The only response I could muster was a weak suggestion that we talk with him together. Even I knew that this would not help.

References

Adler, H. M., and V. B. O. Hammett. 1973. The doctor–patient relationship revisited: an analysis of the placebo effect. *Annals of Internal Medicine* 78:595–98.

Baird, M. A., and W. D. Grant. 1998. Families and health. In R. B. Taylor (ed.). *Family Medicine: Principles and Practice.* 5th ed. New York: Springer, pp. 26–31.

Cassell, E. J. 1976. *The Healer's Art.* Philadelphia: Lippincott.

Christakis, D. A., and C. Feudtner. 1997. Temporary matters: the ethical consequences of transient social relationships in medical training. *Journal of the American Medical Association* 278:739–43.

Fernandez, E. S, J. E. South-Paul, and S. C. Matheny. 1998. Sociocultural Issues in Health Care. In R. B Taylor (ed.). *Family Medicine: Principles and Practice.* 5th ed. New York: Springer, pp. 19–25.

Frank, A. W. 1995. *The Wounded Storyteller: Body, Illness, and Ethics.* Chicago: University of Chicago Press.

Frank, J. 1973. *Persuasion and Healing: A Comparative Study of Psychotherapy.* 2d ed. New York: Schocken.

Helman, C. 1990. *Culture, Health, and Illness: An Introduction for Health Professionals.* 2d ed. Boston: Wright.

Houston, W. R. 1938. The doctor himself as a therapeutic agent. *Annals of Internal Medicine* 11:1416–25.

Huygen, F. J. A. 1978. *Family Medicine: The Medical History of Families.* New York: Brunner/Mazel.

Kleinman, A. F., L. Eisenberg, and B. Good. 1978. Culture, illness and care: clinical lessons from anthropologic and cross-cultural research. *Annals of Internal Medicine* 88:251–58.

Levenstein, J. H., E. C. McCracken, I. R. McWhinney, et al. 1986. The patient-centred clinical method: 1. a model for the doctor–patient interaction in family medicine. *Family Practice* 3:24–30.

Morris, D. B. 1997. Placebo, Pain, and Belief: A Biocultural Model. In A. Harrington (ed.). *The Placebo Effect: An Interdisciplinary Exploration.* Cambridge, Mass.: Harvard University Press, pp. 187–207.

Novack, D. H. 1987. Therapeutic aspects of the clinical encounter. *Journal of General and Internal Medicine* 2:346–55.

Tresolini, C. P., and the Pew-Fetzer Task Force on Advancing Psychosocial Health Education (P-FTF). 1994. Health professions education and relationship-centered care. San Francisco: Pew Health Professions Commission.

Humor

Reflections

Justin Allen and Jeffrey M. Borkan

"Laughter is the best medicine."

The theme of this chapter is humor, particularly the brand attempted by family and general physicians in the stories they write about their clinical experiences. Although physicians are frequently lampooned and satirized, jollity may not fit with our usual notions of "medicine as a serious business." West (1984), who conducted one of the few studies in this area, analyzed audiotaped encounters between fourteen family physician residents and their patients and observed that laughter was uncommon. Health care providers work with the sick, the infirm, and the injured, attempting to heal, or at least relieve suffering. Medicine is one of the most demanding healing professions, requiring high levels of knowledge and skill, long hours of work, and, often, high-stake decisions. The attending high levels of professional stress are themselves reflected in increased rates of suicide, marital breakdown, and alcohol abuse in practitioners (Gerber 1983).

Does all this—both in the art of medicine and later, in narrative representations of clinical encounters—allow humor a role? Our answer is a resounding "Yes!" Humor in many forms helps individuals narrow interpersonal and cultural gaps, express frustration and anger, communicate difficult messages, and cope with anxiety (Wender 1996). Laughter and tears are closely allied as human expressions of emotion, as indeed are the underlying situations of comedy and tragedy. Only a few minor details need to be altered for a tragic situation to become a farce. In addition, medicine, particularly family medicine, is based on interaction between people, and the transaction often has ample potential for jollity, laughter, and fun. The potential benefits are broad, for the patient, the provider, and their relationship.

Benefits to Patients. "Laughter is the best medicine" is an English adage that has long been accepted as true. Indeed, its origin can be traced back to Proverbs 17, verse 22: "A merry heart doeth good like a medicine." There is a broad literature in medicine and nursing on the subject of therapeutic humor. Norman Cousins, a writer who overcame serious illnesses with the help of laughter, helped reopen the subject in the United States in the 1970s and 1980s with lectures, appearances on television and radio talk shows, and popular books (1979; 1989). He equated humor with laughter and saw the potential for a strong therapeutic effect. More recently Erdman (1993), writing on laughter therapy for patients with cancer, suggested that care should be taken to ensure that humor persists even during the bleakest time for patients, families, and medical personnel.

Research has indicated that laughter can lower cortisol levels, a physiologic marker of stress, and influence the function of immunoregulatory cells (Kamei, Kumano, and Masmura, 1997). Squier (1995), who performed a study on humor in the doctor–patient relationship, has suggested that humor can reinforce a sense of equality between physicians and patients. In addition, he found that humor can help build a stronger relationship between them and provides a sense of control and healing for the patient, while not detracting from the patient's perceptions of professional medical care.

Benefits for Doctors. The difficulties of translating a biomedical education to real-life situations of medical practice, particularly in family medicine, has been clearly described by McWhinney (1997). Medical practice is filled with anxiety and uncertainty. To survive we may need to appreciate the funny side of our job, to revel in its occasional ridiculousness, and above all to avoid taking ourselves too seriously. The ability to laugh at one's self may demonstrate both self-awareness and self-esteem. It helps us deal with stress and avoid burnout. Dr. Allen's first introduction to medicine as a "funny business" was in the Richard Gordon's book *Doctor in the House* (1953), which describes the trials and tribulations of medical students and junior doctors. This is an example of a physician laughing at himself and the predicament that faces junior doctors. It also covers the survival mechanisms that they developed to cope with their problems. Its lighthearted view of very stressful periods in physician training was a comfort to Allen's colleagues and him as they struggled with their own equally difficult situations.

Benefits to the Provider–Patient Relationship. A patient who chooses to share an amusing anecdote is granting a great privilege. To cover their embarrassment, patients may invariably precede their revelation by the words "promise not to laugh, but"—something which may be difficult to comply with for the honest provider. However, the ability of physician and patient to share a joke indicates a very powerful doctor–patient relationship. Dr. Allen remembers on one occasion hearing roars of laughter from the consulting room next door, where one of his partners had just confirmed that a patient was pregnant for the fifth time. The woman concerned had said, "I know you'll think this too late, but I've booked an appointment for my husband to see you about a vasectomy." To this physician quipped, "Oh, you've worked out how it's done!"

The authors and the stories in this chapter are very diverse, originating in the United Kingdom, Canada, Israel, and Switzerland. Their humor is often contextually based in local knowledge, yet their appeal is broadly international. The chapter's narratives illustrate a number of different aspects of humor in medicine, but all could have taken place almost anywhere in the world with one or two contextual amendments. For example, Peter Curtis describes how a chance trip to the theater provokes a memory of an early life, when he had to apply his medical skills in very difficult circumstances, which descended to pure farce when surrounded by screaming fans and famous buttocks. Michael Weingarten illustrates the clash between the traditional culture of healing and that of modern medicine. In this story it is the patient who has made the joke.

In two of the other stories, told by Justin Allen and Benedikt Horn, strange circumstances surrounding the events produce the humorous effect. The situations themselves—an acute asthma attack and a panic-inspired hyperventilation problem—are not funny in themselves. The physician-writers were able to appreciate the humor of the situations and to use that to relieve their own stress levels, if not those of their patients. Perle Feldman describes the therapeutic effects of humor, the outcome of making a patient laugh, and the infectious nature of this process.

Are physicians and provider–patient encounters intrinsically funny? Have these clinician-storytellers captured humor in their tales? Perhaps you will be encouraged to believe that providers and patients need to appropriate the therapeutic effect of humor and to learn how to use it in daily encounters. Some contend that primary care providers need to be able to interpret patients' humor, to learn how humor can create a healing environment in order to improve and enrich patient care (Wender 1996). You, the reader, will have to decide, but we hope you will have a few laughs in the meantime!

Once upon a Time in the Land of Rock and Roll

Peter Curtis
London, England

We had just settled into our hotel room after an uneventful flight into London and were quickly skimming the entertainment section of the *Evening Standard* to find a show to go to that night. One of the pleasures of this cultured and fascinating city is to make an impromptu and usually successful choice of a concert or theater, booked at the very last minute—the spontaneity of it all only adding to the enjoyment.

Sipping a cup of burning hot Earl Grey tea brewed in the room, with the entertainment page spread out on the bed, I rapidly scanned past *The Mousetrap* and *Cats*—shows that had been running longer than most people's memories could handle. I was studying the excerpted phrases of acclaim and commentary by well-known drama critics appearing under or above the title of each musical or play. This traditional part of London theater marketing usually provided at least some idea of the quality and content of the show . For instance, "Brilliantly obscure, but diverting" indicated some indigestible avant-garde piece, while "Continues to be irresistibly and funnily slapstick" meant that busloads of visitors and tourists from out of town, even if they didn't understand the language, would be able to laugh at the actors' antics. On the other hand, there were plays that had received the London Theatre Critics' Award, a sign of good quality, and the National Theatre always had something interesting.

Halfway across the entertainment page my skimming came to an abrupt halt at the following words:

WHITEHALL THEATRE
"BEST NEW MUSICAL IN TOWN—BRILLIANT." *2nd rockin' year of the*
ROY ORBISON STORY
Now featuring special guest star PJ PROBY
Last 3 weeks of record-breaking run

It was the name "PJ PROBY" that had caused me to suffer a sudden memory blast, while unintentionally gulping down a mouthful of scalding tea. After all, everyone knew about the glistening black bouffant hair, dark glasses, and almost motionless lips of Roy Orbison singing "Pretty Woman" in the sixties. Who, however, remembered his contemporary, PJ Proby, the rock and roller who split his jeans on stage? PJ was an American boy who had developed his skills duplicating Elvis's pelvic gyrations. He had a following in Europe, especially England, rather than in the States. This was probably because, in the permissive "swinging sixties" of England, the splitting of jeans to show certain areas of youthful flesh in public was not only acceptable but positively thrilling—while in the United States it was still immoral.

The reason for my shock was that PJ, who was now probably around fifty, was a distant acquaintance of mine. We had once had a chance encounter in the course of each other's duties, mine as a physician just out of training and his as an up and-coming rock and roll star. At the time he was playing to jam-packed audiences of teenagers at the London Palladium, one of the city's biggest theaters, while I was busy with two jobs. I was a senior resident doing a urology rotation at a teaching hospital during the day then working for a medical service at night. As I sat on the hotel bed, reminiscing, I could not easily recall his features, but I distinctly remembered the circumstances of our meeting and many details about his body below waist level.

I moonlighted at a "deputizing" medical service, a commercial enterprise that offered general practitioners in London an escape from both serious and frivolous night calls. The British National Health Service required that all family physicians be available to their registered patients for emergencies and house calls after normal working hours, but how this was organized was up to them. The company for which I worked, or perhaps "slaved" is a better term, used inexperienced hospital residents and a number of offbeat physicians who could not get work elsewhere as deputies, to provide this after-hours care. This was at low cost to the GPs, who were able to get a good night's sleep knowing that their patients would at least be seen that night. We were paid a flat fee for a twelve-hour shift with a bonus if we handled more than twenty calls. No additional payment could be accepted from patients, even if they offered Although it was exhausting, the second job helped to pay the rent for my newly started family.

A small central base, staffed by two clerks, communicated by radiotelephone with the roving doctors who made the calls. We drove around the city in Austin minis, oversized tin cracker boxes on tiny wheels, brilliantly designed to be economical and easy to park. (I also believed that the Greek born engineer who designed this tiny but very fashionable car was taking subtle revenge on the tall Anglo-Saxons who had stolen large pieces of the Acropolis in the last century and put them in the British Museum.) The minis were usually on their last legs, their gearboxes mangled by innumerable half-asleep doctors and their bodywork dented and twisted from many a bump in the night.

We were equipped with a small medical bag full of pharmaceutical samples, a blood pressure cuff, some dressings, syringes, needles, prescription pads, a flashlight, and, of course, a detailed map of the city. The calls came in over the radio, usually giving us some idea of the problem and the name and address of the patient. Most were the straightforward primary care problems of otitis media (middle ear infections), common colds, diarrhea, headaches, high fever, and "the miseries." Of course, in a city like London there were always strange and mysterious episodes to be experienced, such as being chased down a street by an axe-wielding psychotic or trying to dig a West Indian family out from under a collapsed ceiling in their rented room. These gave the long, tiring and miserably paid nights a bit of excitement and glamor.

Every once in a while I would be given a section of London that included the entertainment district and a number of big hotels. This often added more unusual social situations and medical problems to the standard night call menu, and it was on one of those nights that I met PJ Proby. The call came through from base control that a man urgently needed a doctor to give him an injection at the Mayfair Hotel—one of the most prestigious establishments in the city. The deputizing service was covering the practice of the hotel doctor, who was safely in bed somewhere across town. Unfortunately the clerks did not know the patient's name or the problem—only that it was on the top floor of the hotel.

I pushed the mini as hard as it would go, wondering what an "urgent injection" implied and how sick this patient was likely to be. I imagined that it was probably some diabetic control problem to do with insulin. A pity, because I didn't have any insulin in the bag. In about fifteen minutes the tin box on wheels sputtered to a halt just behind an impeccable cream-colored Rolls-Royce resting outside the magnificent entrance to the hotel. This was guarded by an equally magnificent very large doorman wearing a suede tophat, a waxed moustache, and a uniform dripping with gold braid that jangled when he moved. I got out of the car with my medical bag and immediately told the doorman about the patient on the top floor in urgent need of an injection. "I don't know nuffin' about a man needin' an injection," he said, eyeing my wrinkled clothes and the pitiable machine that had brought me there, "and anyway, mate, yer can't leave that blinkin' heap in front of the 'otel." But my dedication to healing the sick proved even stronger than my shame at the way this giant ex–army drill sergeant looked at my transport and me. "You park it then!" I said. As I rushed into the lobby, I called out, "And be careful with it—its a special medical call car."

The lobby was busy with well-dressed guests getting ready to go to concerts, dinner, or the theater. However, in addition I saw many clusters of adolescents, most of them girls, talking excitedly and darting about between the marble pillars. Closer inspection revealed that the majority wore sweaters bearing the imprinted words "PJ Proby Fan Club." Of course, I had seen him on television and presumed that he was staying at the hotel.

With my attention refocused on the urgent call, I strode up to the reception desk and told the clerk who I was and why I had come. "Oh, yes!" he said, "We've been expecting you. Please wait here and Mr. Jablonsky will be down in a minute."

Within moments, a short, round, balding, cigar-puffing man, wearing a blazing tie surrounded by a white suit, came bustling up to me. " Hi doc!" he said, " I'm PJ's manager and am I sure glad you've come! He's goin' on stage in twennie minutes. Come on up—we've gotta hurry!" He took me by the elbow, steered me away from the lobby, and took me along a number of passages till we reached a small service elevator. He and I just managed to squeeze into it. "We gotta keep outta the way of those goddam' fans," he grunted. "They always find ways to grab hold of PJ. By the way, Doc, yew got yore syringes with yew?" It was then I realized that PJ was the patient in urgent need of an injection.

We entered PJ's suite after Mr. Jablonsky had given a coded knock on the door. At the far end of the room, several people were clustered around the star. He was wearing a shimmering shirt and velveteen pants and stood absolutely still. As we approached, I noticed that a middle-aged woman with a sewing basket on her knees was sitting on a stool beside him, threading a needle. Watched by the other members of the entourage, she was performing a most delicate task—sewing PJ snugly into his jeans in such a way that he could, at the exactly prescribed moment on stage, rotate his hips and split open the seams.

While I watched with professional interest, Mr. Jablonsky had pulled out a cardboard box, slipped off the lid, and handed me a twenty–cubic centimeter glass vial of murky greenish fluid. "These are essential vitamins," he said. "PJ gets a shot ever' night, just before he goes on stage—keeps him goin' night after night." He paused, "Don't worry yourself, Doc, we get these shots from PJ's doc in the States—it's all legal, so just get on with it. We ain't got much time and this is his last show in London!"

I got the syringe and needle ready, cracked open the vial, and drew up the rather viscous fluid. I approached PJ from behind while he turned his head and half acknowledged me. After all, he probably got this from a different doctor every night—with no opportunity to build up the doctor–patient relationship. But I was faced with a dilemma. PJ was already sewn tightly into his pants, so I had the option of plunging the needle through the velveteen into his buttock or asking for the thread to be undone to expose his bare flesh. I chose the latter route and, with a sigh, my seamstress colleague bent to her task of undoing PJ.

At that very moment, someone in the corridor used the coded knock and the door was opened. With yelps of triumph, six teenage girls wearing PJ sweaters rushed into the room delighted to have found the inner sanctum but not expecting to see him standing there in full frontal splendor with his pants below his knees. Their reaction was a mixture of shrieking, sobbing, leaping about, and near fainting. While Mr. Jablonsky and the others rushed to deal with the crisis, I quickly plunged the needle into PJ's buttock and steadily forced the energy-giving fluid into him. No sooner done than my colleague rapidly and dextrously used her finer needle to sew the maroon velveteen back into its buttock-hugging shape. PJ Proby was ready to take on the London audience at last.

On my way out of the suite, I briefly checked the ecstatic fans to make sure that they had recovered their jubilant adolescent apoplexy, and found that all was well. They would have a wonderful story to tell their parents.

Mr. Jablonsky accompanied me down in the service elevator, puffing on his cigar. "That was a tough situation, Doc!" he said. "Yew took care of it real good. Do yew think this will handle it?" He pulled out a wad of pound notes and thrust them into my breast pocket, just the way I had seen it done in the movies. I thought of telling Mr. Jablonsky about the rules of the deputizing service—no cash payments. On the other hand, this was PJ's last appearance in London for a while, so probably no one would find out about my illicit fee. So I thanked him, found my way to the lobby, and departed through the revolving door at the front of the hotel.

After the doorman had arranged for my mini to be brought out from where he had been hiding it, I pulled a couple of pound notes from my breast pocket and thanked him.

My wife called to me from the bathroom in our room, bringing me into the present with a jolt. "So, have you chosen a show for us to go to, Peter ? You've been staring at the newspaper long enough!"

I wondered what PJ Proby would be doing on stage as a guest star in the Roy Orbison story—surely not what he had done every night thirty years ago—and I did not intend to find out. "Just can't make my mind up," I called back.

Epilogue

There is a certain circularity to our lives that is often undetected in the uneven linear experience of daily work and play. It is odd how people and events come out of the past to haunt you and give pleasure—students you taught, babies you delivered, people you joked with, villages you visited. As doctors, we are lucky that we have so many people who knew us in the terrible and wonderful moments of their lives.

Healers: The Physician and the Mori

Michael Weingarten
Rosh Haayan, Israel

I was thirty-three; she was sixty-six. I had been in my new practice for six months and Naomi had been to see me at least a dozen times already. Hers was one of the few faces I could put a name to. She had come to Israel from the Yemen in 1950, flying through the darkness of a clandestine airlift. Overnight she crossed the centuries between the medieval culture of her childhood and the modernity of her new and progressive young state.

Her file was fat with tests which failed to solve the enigma of her recurrent abdominal cramps. I told her I thought it pointless to order any more. She was silent but looked relieved. "What now?" I ventured. "I don't know," she replied. I asked if she had been to the mori (a traditional Yemenite Jewish rabbi–healer). She had, of course, but had been shy to talk to me about it. Actually, she said, the mori wanted me, the doctor, to write him a note to say that he could go ahead with his treatment. He wanted to give her makweh over all the upper part of her body. I knew all about makweh by now; 70 percent of my Yemenite patients had scars from this healing method— branding by red hot iron nails. They had it for sciatica on the side of the ankle; for renal colic—in the loin; for impotence—on the forehead. I thought it was an admirable caution of the mori to check with me first, so I wrote the note for Naomi, who was looking quite apprehensive. "Do you think it'll help?" I asked.

"I don't really know, Doctor," she answered. "In the Yemen it certainly would have worked, but here, in Israel, God has taken the right to heal away from the mori, and He has given it to you, the doctors. But you're not so good at it."

Magic and Technology

Justin Allen
Leicestershire, United Kingdom

The phone rang at 2 A.M.—or, rather, the phone blasted a noise akin to an electric alarm clock. So I drowsily took what seemed to be the best course of action and turned off the alarm. The noise persisted.

My wife woke up (which is unusual—she sleeps through most of my night calls, a fact which I find quite unreasonably infuriating). "It's the phone," she said helpfully. I picked up the bedside phone and after struggling in the dark to find the right button, turned it on. There was only a dial tone, and the alarm noise persisted.

I think less clearly than I used to, particularly at that time of night. Long gone are the days, if they ever existed, when I used to leap excitedly from my bed to rush off and save another life. I sat holding the telephone, pondering the fact that something was still ringing; having apparently run out of options, I was idly wondering what to do.

"Not that one—the practice phone," she said. We had recently purchased a superneat pocket-sized cellular phone, which was somewhere on the bedside table. However, these things have a life of their own and can move from where you left them while your back is turned. I frequently have to resort to calling myself to find out where it has got to. On this occasion I couldn't find it, so I turned on the light, knocking over a glass of water in the process. I finally located the phone, and, sitting on the edge of the bed with my feet in a puddle of icy water, I managed to answer it.

Things did not get any better: "Can you come? He's gone green and is barking like a dog."

Some of the water had obviously got into the phone and was distorting the sound. "Could you repeat that?" I asked.

"Its my husband—he's gone green and he's barking like a dog. Can you come and see him?"

My brain was having a little problem dealing with this information. "Sorry," I said, without thinking. She started to repeat the message. "No, I heard you," I interrupted, "but I don't really understand. Can you tell me a bit more about the problem?"

"Well, I just woke up and heard him making this funny noise while breathing, and he can't talk to me. He seems ever so ill. . . ." At this point she started to cry. I took down the name and address and told her I was on my way, suggesting that she lay him on his side—it seemed like a good idea at the time.

I got dressed loudly, as I always do, in the hope that somebody else in the house would wake up and be sympathetic. As usual, they all slept on. Again, I was mildly irrationally perturbed, and I left the silent house. I set off in the car rehearsing possible clinical scenarios. A form of convulsion perhaps, or maybe a stroke? Or could this be an acute psychotic episode? I could see myself spending all night on the call if that were the case!

The family lived in a village about six miles away, and I had to drive along narrow country roads to get there. I was about a mile or so short of my destination when the phone sounded again. In the good old days, before cellular phones, there was never the problem of answering the phone when driving. This is a highly developed skill that I do not possess. The first problem is picking it up in the dark the right way up, and the second is to find the "on" button. After several trips onto the grass berm, and a skirmish or two with hedgerows, I have decided that driving and phoning do not mix. I remain envious of those who I see driving along motorways apparently shaving and answering the phone simultaneously!

I stopped the car, found the phone, and answered it. It was the brother of my "barking" patient. "I'm ringing on behalf of my brother. My sister-in-law just rang for a visit. We were wondering how long you would be?"

This is an entirely new hazard of the communication technology explosion. On several occasions I have had to stop on my way to a call to answer requests for progress reports! For some reason this does not improve my temper. I assured him that I would arrive sooner if I did not have to keep stopping to answer such queries.

I arrived at the house to find panic well established. Jane, the original caller, was crouching on the floor of the bedroom, crying. David, the patient, was lying face down on the bed. His parents and his brother, who live on adjacent streets, had been summoned and were milling around downstairs. The brother, who for good measure had brought his wife and baby with him, met me at the car. He proceeded to drag the door open and hurried me into the house, muttering helpful things about calling ambulances.

A quick glance at David was all that was needed to confirm that he was in tetany[1] from overbreathing. He had classical carpopedal spasm and was taking breaths in frequent noisy gasps. They did not sound doglike to me, but this was the noise that concerned the family. His green color was a result of the lampshade on the only available light in the bedroom, which was at the bedside. It was fitted with a very low power bulb, so that whole scene was in a sort of surrealistic gloom.

During my training I had been taught that this problem was best dealt with by the rebreathing of expired air from a large paper bag. I asked the

---

1. Tetany is a disorder marked by intermittent tonic muscular contractions, tremors, paresthesias, and muscle pain. It can be caused by rapid or forced breathing which reduces the carbon dioxide in the blood. A typical sympton is carpopedal spasm, which refers to the hands (or wrists) and the feet.

family to find me one. However, in our modern throwaway society everything is packed in polyethylene bags, and nobody uses paper. There is a problem using polyethylene bags in this situation. Having been taught from their mother's knee that you can be suffocated by polyethylene bags, patients and their relatives can rarely be convinced that you are acting in their best interests when you place a plastic bag over the mouth and nose of someone with apparent breathing difficulties.

My request for a large paper bag caused complete uproar. Downstairs a sotto voce discussion was going on about what they should do about the doctor going mad. Upstairs a frantic search was under way, with much turning out of drawers and cupboards. Meanwhile I had managed to persuade the patient to slow up on the barking and calm his breathing a bit. I ascertained what had happened. The whole family had been vomiting with a sickness and diarrhea bug, and he had wakened feeling sick. His mother had always told him that he could overcome this feeling by taking deep breaths. He had duly tried this, a bit too vigorously, and the rest was history, so to speak.

Eventually, after much rummaging, a large brown envelope was found and put to work, with very satisfying results. The patient sat up and pronounced himself better, and Jane stopped crying, but she seemed shaken by the whole experience. Under these circumstances I often resort to saying, "It's all right now, you can put the life insurance policies away, he's going to live," as a way of easing tension. I tried it.

My reputation as a magician was made forever! "How did you know?" she gasped. She held up the papers that she had removed from the now soggy envelope before we had used it, to display the logo of a well-known insurance company. "It was the only envelope I could find."

She Laughed

Perle Feldman
Montreal, Quebec

Sue Jong was a young Chinese commercial artist born in Hong Kong. She had been living in Canada for quite some time. Her English was good but her husband's was less so. When she was in her thirty sixth week of pregnancy she told me that her mother was coming from Hong Kong to be with her at the time of birth and to help her with the baby. "She wants to bring me all kinds of Chinese medicines, but I know I can't take those," Sue said sadly. "Do you want to take them? " I asked. Shyly, she nodded. "Then why not?" Sue then explained to me that she thought I would disapprove of her using Chinese traditional medicines, and she did not want me to be angry. I explained to her that I had a lot of respect for the thousands of years of tradition behind Chinese herbal medicine; as long as it did not interfere with the stuff I was doing, I did not mind at all.

When the time of the birth came, Sue had a long, slow labor. Steven Tsui, the resident,[2] spoke Cantonese well enough to communicate with the husband and the patient's mother. We called for an epidural[3] and William Khazzar, one of my first clinical teachers, came to administer it. I was pleased and surprised to see him, since he had just moved to this hospital. Dr. Khazzar always combined a real concern for both students and patients with a low-key, incisive humor. The epidural he inserted was a dream. It relieved the pain while still allowing the patient to move around and push effectively.

She was fully dilated an hour later. When her pain was relieved, Steve asked her about the medicines her mother had brought from Hong Kong. Sue told us that her mother had brought a special Korean ginseng wine, which was supposed to be taken just as the head was crowning.[4] Steven was impressed: "Wow—real Korean ginseng." We assured Sue that we would try and help her take it at just the right time. She soon began to push, as her husband supported her. The chemistry in the room was happy and positive, not too much noise. She pushed the head down to the perineum and soon it began to crown. I waited. The head crowned a bit more, but still I waited.

"Aren't you going to cut an episiotomy?" Marie-Elana, the nurse, asked me. "Nope," I said. Even though the head, which was still crowning, had

---

2. A resident is a doctor who has completed the intern year and is assigned as house officer to a particular hospital for clinical training.

3. An epidural is pain medication administered outside the sac (dura) covering the spinal cord.

4. Crowning is the stage of childbirth where the baby's head has negotiated the pelvic outlet and is stretching the vulva.

been stretching Sue's perineum for more than ten minutes, the patient had experienced no pain. Her perineum was long and tough, and the baby's heartbeat was fine. I wanted to wait.

"Tch! You'll never get it out without a tear," Marie-Elana stated emphatically, making a sound West Indians use to express disbelief. "Is that a bet?" I asked. "You're on," said Marie-Elana.

"Move over," I said to Steven, "I'm afraid I have to do this one." At the same time I sent up a little silent prayer, "Please, please don't let me get into trouble for showing off." My patient thought this whole interchange was funny; she started to giggle. Her husband whispered something into her ear. She started to laugh out loud. Somehow that laughter produced the right combination of pressure and relaxation. The baby's brow began to slip over the edge of the perineum.

"Quick, take your ginseng," I said, "and keep laughing." This must have sounded really silly; both the patient and her husband burst into laughter. It was infectious. Soon we were all laughing and giggling helplessly, while the baby's head slipped gently over the perineum as I guided and slowed it. This child was born as every person in the room was laughing. He cried briefly and reassuringly, turning pink and rosy.

"So?" Marie-Elana said to me. I inspected the patient's perineum as Sue inspected her baby's fingers and toes. I grinned in triumph. "Not a scratch." Afterwards, as we were doing the paperwork, Marie-Elana approached me. "You know, that was a beautiful delivery."

"Yes," said Steven. "I'm going to remember this one." "So will I," I said.

Epilogue

For me, the best deliveries are those where "nothing happens." Unlike many of my obstetrical colleagues, I am not thrilled by difficult and complicated cases. What interests me are people's lives and how they deal with what is happening to them. The most uneventful births can sometimes be the most satisfying.

I remember this birth because I had such a good time doing it.

William Tell and Me: A General Practitioner on Stage

Benedikt P. Horn

Interlaken, Switzerland

When the German poet Friedrich Schiller finished his drama *Wilhelm Tell* (William Tell), he had no idea that it would become the Swiss national drama. Interlaken, in the heart of Switzerland, is the place where Schiller's *Tell* has been performed twenty times annually for the last eighty-four years, on a splendid natural stage with platform seating for about two thousand spectators. The actors are enthusiastic amateurs, and about twenty horses and a large cast of cows and goats take part as well. I played the title role of William Tell for seven years and experienced some interesting medical problems on stage—including some personal dramas.

When the performance begins, visitors from around the world can admire an extraordinary autumnal return from the Alps of cows, horses, and goats — a unique scene in the world of theater. A few years ago, I suffered from stress and stage fright just before the opening scene when I was to appear as William Tell for the first time that season. Just as I readied for my appearance, a first-aid layman ran up to me and cried "Doctor, come immediately, a young lady spectator is dying." William Tell knew that he had to be on stage in three or four minutes and suggested calling the emergency doctor.

Despite my protestations, one minute later the head of the first-aid team dragged me to the emergency room, crying that the woman would die without me. Duty calls— my profession is more important than the role I have to play. A young newlywed from New Zealand lies on the stretcher, blue from asphyxia, apneic, and deeply comatose. I put down my crossbow and begin immediately with cardiopulmonary resuscitation (CPR). I hear the cattle passing with their large and loud cowbells . . . two minutes left and I am due on stage. While performing CPR, I wonder who could continue for me. I think of another general practitioner in the cast: "Call Doctor B. immediately!"

My colleague plays the part of a priest and is already dressed in his costume complete with the crucifix in one hand. When he enters the emergency room the patient's husband collapses and groans, "No priest, no priest!" The "priest" continues with CPR and some seconds later I am on stage, not as a doctor but as William Tell with my crossbow, ready to speak my first lines.

The performance was saved and so was the patient and her husband. After spending two days in the intensive care unit, she was discharged from hospital and was able to carry on with her honeymoon.

William Tell was not a politician, but he was always ready to help when the community needed him. Similarities between general practitioners and William Tell are purely coincidental.

References

Cousins, N. 1979. Anatomy of an Illness as Perceived by the Patient. New York: Norton.

Cousins, N. 1989. *The Laughter Connection: Head First: The Biology of Hope and the Healing Power of the Spirit.* New York: Penguin Books.

Erdman, L. 1993. Laughter therapy for patients with cancer. *Journal of Psycho-social Oncology.* 11(4):55–67.

Gerber, L. A. 1983. *Married to Their Careers.* New York: Tavistock.

Gordon, R. 1953. *Doctor in the House.* New York: Harcourt Brace.

Kamei, T., H. Kumano, and S. Masmura. 1997. Changes in immunoregulatory cells associated with psychological stress and humor. *Perceptual and Motor Skills* 84: 1296–98.

McWhinney, I. R. 1997. *A Textbook of Family Medicine.* New York: Oxford University Press.

Squier, H. A. 1995. Humor in the doctor/patient relationship. *Family Systems Medicine* 13:101–7.

Wender, R. C. 1996. Humor in medicine. *Primary Care* 23(1):141–54.

West, C. 1984. Laughter and sociable commentary in medical encounters. In C. West (ed.). *Routine Complications: Troubles with Talk between Doctors and Patients.* Bloomington: Indiana University Press.

Abuse

Reflections

Carol P. Herbert and Shmuel Reis

Is there family violence among my patients? Are there adult survivors of child-hood abuse—sexual, physical, emotional—or neglect? Are the media and the medical social science literature correct in reporting abuse rates that may in-clude a quarter or more of the adult population? Family physicians worldwide ask themselves these questions (Mammen and Olsen 1996). The three stories in this chapter seem to support this contention.

These stories (as well as two in Chapter 9, "Tincture of Time" and "Un-resolved Grief") simultaneously reflect the mythology that continues to sur-round family violence while portraying how family physicians can learn to pro-mote healing. What is known is that family violence, including sexual abuse, crosses socioeconomic, cultural, and religious lines (Cohen, De Vos, and Newberger 1997). Its high prevalence among adults is quite stable in almost every country and social group in which it has been investigated (Mazza, Dennerstein, and Ryan 1996). Family violence is a major source of psychopa-thology in later years, not infrequently manifesting in vague physical com-plaints (Buist 1995). Boys are affected (Antao et al. 1996), but females are in-volved to a larger extent. Sometimes physicians come across sexual abuse through gynecological complaints or symptoms (Kirkengen, Schei, and Steine 1993). Obtaining board certification in family medicine doesn't guarantee effective care of abused patients (Tudiver, Permaul, and Woods 1996), and there is still much room for improvement in the medical profession's aware-ness and therapeutic interventions in victims of abuse.

Many themes relating to abuse are dealt with in the accounts in this chapter. Hava Tabenkin experiences the shock that many practitioners have suffered: the utter disbelief that this could happen here, to my patients, in my community. She is confronted with the power relationships that are part of the reality of sexual abuse. "Consent" becomes irrelevant in the face of a relationship with huge power differentials, whether this is between parent and child, older sibling and younger sibling, or between a six-year-old and a thirteen-year-old boy. Implicit here too is the myth that "boys will be boys," downplaying the evident impact on the abused.

In Judith Hollis–Triantafillou's story of Katerina, the myth that "trivial" abuse or neglect is of no consequence is exposed. Katerina tells of her sterile relationship with her mother as a child: since she could do no right, her only recourse was to rebel as an adolescent and to escape her family home by way of an early marriage. Her multiple physical symptoms and emotional distress are common outcomes of childhood abuse and neglect. To the young child, feeling unloved or invisible is devastating to self-esteem. It is only as an adult that Katerina realizes the extent of her deprivation, which she had repressed.

John Gunzburg's disturbing story demonstrates how victims believe themselves to be responsible for their abuse, accepting the lies told by the abuser. Sonja "hides" in hobnailed boots and jeans, "her hair tied tightly behind her head," fearful of drawing sexual attention. She has no sense of safety in personal relationships; her lack of trust and inner rage are turned outward in her obsession with knives, reinforcing her view of herself as "evil-natured" and dangerous.

Keeping the secret of child abuse is a behavior fostered by abusers and supported by families and communities. Abusers avoid punishment by convincing children like Sonja and Ron not to tell, threatening them with the sometimes sadly accurate assurance that they will be blamed. Families and communities convince themselves that to expose the abuse will compound the trauma; it is better to go on as though nothing had happened. Unfortunately for many child victims, this denial of their reality, the betrayal of their trust, and the violation of their physical and psychological boundaries compounds the damage. Dr. Tabenkin wonders correctly: "How will [Danny] know his deeds were wrong?" "How will Ron recognize that what was done to him was immoral if the perpetrator is not punished?" Neither child victim nor perpetrator is well served by denial—sensitive treatment of both children can be better managed in a context of honesty and openness. An opportunity was lost to educate these children and others on the kibbutz about conduct in relationships and abuses of power.

The most effective model in such situations may be to hold the perpetrator responsible in order to assist him to acknowledge responsibility for his behavior so that he recognizes his capacity to choose to behave differently. Thus blame and punishment are less the issue than moral responsibility.

The three stories speak to family physicians about our opportunities and obligations (Herbert 1991) to intervene in situations of abuse. Dr. Hollis-Triantafillou's index of suspicion and unconditional offer to listen to Katerina and Dr. Gunzburg's willingness to engage with Sonja and look beyond the facade allow their patients to disclose painful truths. We see evidence of healing in both stories, fostered by a safe patient–physician relationship. Conversely, Dr. Tabenkin, in courageously exposing her own failure to diagnose the psychosocial basis of biological symptoms in her patients, is in good company. The literature is replete with stories of battered women medicated for depression; "bad" adolescents jailed or left in their abusive families; "perfect" children and adults who fear that their secret will be discovered and that they will be blamed unless they maintain their masks. Family physicians need to remind themselves that disclosures are not easy for survivors, many of whom do not identify themselves as victimized. The family physician must look carefully at the signs and symptoms and ask questions that are at once clear and gentle, allowing the survivor to tell her or his story.

We can all learn from Dr. Gunzburg, whose modeling of a respectful, caring relationship reflects his sensitivity to the exquisite vulnerability of sexual abuse survivors in relationships with therapists. He courageously acknowledges that he is sexually aroused in the intimate relationship with Sonja and declares the responsibility of the therapist neither to act on his feelings nor to react to the neediness of survivors for warmth and love. His description of the violin serenade is a metaphor for unconditional love and caring, which had profound impact on his patient.

We learn also from Dr. Gunzburg that victims need us as physicians to be nonjudgmental toward them, to be steady in our support, during their healing process. That Dr. Gunzburg could listen unflinchingly to Sonja's fantasies of murder and dismemberment allowed her to discharge her rage safely. Sonja declared her transformation from victim to survivor by figuratively punishing her abusers rather than continuing to blame herself. We have heard such horror fantasies from both children and adults as they face the ugliness of their family pasts.

We are also reminded by Sonja's story of the risks to the physician who may be "vicariously traumatized" by hearing the stories of abuse (McCann and Pearlman 1990). Physicians who have themselves been victimized may have unfinished emotional business which prevents their engaging with abused patients. Only by distancing and denial of their patients' distress can they deny their own pain. There are also physicians whose vulnerability, because of their own losses or unresolved pain, leads them to engage sexually with a patient, a morally indefensible act. However, we must realize that there are physicians who are frankly predatory, who abuse their power in patient–physician relationships to gratify themselves sexually. The profession must police itself to root out such abusers, who recapitulate the abuse that their patient has suffered in childhood and compound the damage.

In summary, the patient–primary care physician's relationship provides a venue for healing. As physicians we must be open to the possibility that any of our patients may have been victimized; we must ask questions fearlessly and wait patiently for our patients to feel safe enough to tell their stories. Our modeling of a nonsexual, caring relationship between equals allows patients to practice a different way of relating, which they can carry over to their social relationships. While only a few of us will have special training and commitment to provide psychotherapy, all family physicians must be prepared to provide medical care to survivors of abuse. In primary care, we have particular opportunity because of the longitudinal nature of our relationships with patients to diagnose abuse and manage its consequences, thus breaking the intergenerational cycle of abuse (Rosenberg et al. 1997). It is both our opportunity and our obligation.

Revenge Is Sweet

Judith Hollis-Triantafillou
Athens, Greece

She'd been lurking for some time in a corner of the waiting room, giving up her turn to two other patients and a drug rep,[1] before finally presenting herself before me right at the end of a long Friday evening surgery. I was not altogether surprised to see her and indeed had partly provoked the visit when I saw her daughter Eirini the previous week.

Eirini had been a patient of mine for three years and was usually accompanied on her visits by her father. I did not know the family well but I had the impression that he was actually her step-father; Eirini was a rather solemn twelve year old with a guarded expression, and he always took great care of her, doing his best to make her laugh and generally behaving very affectionately toward her. But was he perhaps too affectionate? Was I missing something here? I had checked the family records for details, finding them incomplete, and had made a note to investigate further on her next visit.

So when Eirini arrived last week with her mother for her second hepatitis vaccination, I made a few more inquiries and found that the parents were indeed divorced, her natural father living on a distant island where Eirini spent her summers. The new "father" had lived for several years in what was described as a stable relationship with her mother, although they were not in fact married. Gentle probing revealed nothing much further; they all seemed happy enough together but I had the definite impression that the mother was holding something back. I therefore spent a few extra moments chatting with her and Eirini, making sure they both understood that I was available to either of them should they wish to see me alone at any time. And now here she was, visiting me for the first time as a patient: a dark, overweight, anxious-looking woman with a sheaf of medical investigations in her hand and a long story to tell me.

Her name was Katerina and she was thirty-six years old. She'd been generally unwell for four or five years with numerous vague physical complaints, a gradual weight gain, and difficulty sleeping. Visits to a succession of specialists had produced no definite diagnosis, although last year she'd been given thyroid hormone on what I considered to be insufficient evidence that her thyroid gland was not working. More recently her symptoms had been gynecological, recurrent vaginal yeast infection being diagnosed and mildly impaired glucose tolerance (which could mean predisposition to diabetes)

---

1. A drug rep is a sales representative for pharmaceutical companies (a detail man or woman).

discovered on further investigation. There was a strong family history of diabetes, so maybe this was the cause of all her troubles. I took a dietary history, which was appalling: she drank about six cups of heavily sweetened coffee at work each day supplemented by cheese pies and cookies before coming home to cook a meal for the three of them, then more coffee and sugary snacks during the evening. She'd also smoked at least two packs of cigarettes daily for the past fifteen years.

I examined her; she was twenty-five kilos (about fifty-five pounds) overweight with a rapid pulse, moderately high blood pressure, and a smoker's chest. There were no other abnormal findings and, specifically, no signs of thyroid disease. She dressed and we discussed the situation. I explained that whatever the underlying diagnosis, the first step was to stop smoking, exercise, and lose weight, and I made some suggestions as to how this could be achieved. "I don't think I can do it," she said rather helplessly. "Why not?" "I've got problems." "What problems?"

I waited and as the tears began to fall pushed the box of tissues closer to her across the desk. After crying for some minutes she blew her nose, apologized—"I know I'm behaving like a child"—and began to tell me about her mother.

The second of two children, her older brother had always been his mother's darling while Katerina could seemingly do no right in her mother's eyes. She described a childhood during which she was unable to recall a single act of spontaneous affection from her mother toward herself and, like many children in such situations, had assumed the fault to be hers. She tried desperately to conform to what her mother seemed to demand of her—always, of course, without success. Her father, she said, had loved her but his rather ineffectual attempts to support Katerina had only provoked more jealous tantrums from her mother. He had died quite suddenly five years previous to that office visit.

Katerina's eventual rebellion during her younger years caused the situation at home to deteriorate still further, and she eventually escaped to a hasty marriage which had ended in divorce shortly after the birth of her daughter, Eirini. With a baby to care for and no means of support, she'd been forced to turn again to her parents; her mother flatly refused to have her back in the house, reluctantly agreeing instead to look after the child while Katerina found a job.

Strangely enough it was only then, working in a busy office with a dozen or so other women, that she began to be aware for the first time of the extent of her deprivation. A solitary child, school friends not welcomed at home, and later on, struggling alone to cope with the problems of everyday life, she'd had little time to reflect on her own situation. Now the chatter of the other women, constantly discussing their families, had suddenly made her painfully aware of what she had missed out on. The complete picture was so depressing that I felt I really must try to find at least one small spark of joy to brighten the gloom, but, apart from her currently good relationship with her ex-husband, there seemed to be none.

"And another thing," she went on, "All through my childhood I really longed for and begged to be allowed to have a dog."

Her mother had hated all animals and claimed to be allergic to dogs. "You could have one now," I suggested rather tentatively. For the first time that evening a hint of a smile showed on her face.

"I've already got one—we bought it for Eirini, a lovely little terrier called David, so affectionate and no trouble at all." She paused and her smile broadened. "The funny thing is that he absolutely hates my mother. Whenever she goes past in the hallway or he hears her in the garden he goes mad, barking like a maniac and leaping up at her in a frenzy. She's terrified of him and keeps telling me to keep him shut in the house but somehow I always forget and leave the door open and when he starts barking I hide behind the door urging him on !"

We were both laughing by now as she stood up to go, making another appointment to see me in two weeks time. Driving home that evening, still chuckling over the picture of the little dog David yapping away defiantly at Goliath, I felt hopeful that the first step had been taken on the long road back to good family health.

Music to Her Ears

John C. Gunzburg
Victoria, Australia

It was January 1992. My family practice is structured so that I am able to provide weekly forty-minute sessions to some of my patients. Sonja, a thirty-one-year-old gardener, came to me after her previous therapist of nine years had died from a heart attack. Sonja felt that she had killed him, poisoning him with her evil nature.

As it happened great evils had been perpetrated on Sonja during her childhood, including sexual abuse by her father, William, who had died from a heart attack six years previously; lack of protection and complete denial of the abuse from her mother, Elspeth; and discounting and negativity by most members within her extended family. Sonja had indeed herself been poisoned!

For the first six months of weekly therapy (each encounter lasting forty minutes), Sonja came to sessions dressed in shirts with sleeves rolled up, wearing jeans and big hobnailed boots, and with her hair tied tightly behind her head. Her message to me seemed to be quite clear: "Get too close to me, buster, and I will stomp all over you!"

We talked about Sonja's obsession with knives. Because she experienced murderous thoughts toward all her friends and lovers, she had locked away carefully all knives in her kitchen. Sonja was terrified that one day she would stab a companion to death.

Yet behind her tough facade, Sonja occasionally let me glimpse brief flashes of a warm, tender, and fun-loving interior. About six months into therapy, I commented: "I hope one day you will let me see your soft, sensitive side." Sonja shuddered visibly.

Over the next six months we discussed the nature of relationships: negotiating, sharing, arranging closeness and distance, and the fair handling of power. Sonja agreed to collect all the knives that she did not need (enormous butcher's knives and all!) and put them in the dustbin on collection night. This she did. I also placed a fairly blunt letter opener on the chair next to her in the therapy room, and every few weeks replaced it with a sharper blade, in an attempt to desensitize Sonja to the fear of her using it lethally.

Eventually Sonja and I participated together in the ritual burning of a family photograph—the family that had participated in the sham of her "happy childhood." She scattered the ashes to sea off the local pier. This act seemed to have an impact. About six weeks later, Sonja attended our session dressed in a multicolored pastel blouse and lilac skirt, her hair down in long flowing tresses, and wearing lipstick. I felt touched, even privileged, and said: "Sonja, today you have given me a gift, something very special, a treasure that you do not easily share with others. Today, I am going to give you something special in return." I happened to have my violin in my car ready for a performance at a charity concert that evening. I brought it into the therapy room, and played Sonja a medley of Hebrew and Gypsy melodies.

Sonja flipped! "Wow, Dr. John," she said, "'that was wonderful! I feel as though you have serenaded me."

"And of course I have," I responded quietly. "And wouldn't it have been lovely if your Dad had behaved as appropriately toward you when you were a child when he felt his attraction toward you?"

As therapy proceeded, Sonja described how, when making love, she often considered stabbing her lovers full of holes. I commented that sometimes when people are sexually abused as children, the "wiring gets confused and sex and anger get all mixed up." I encouraged Sonja to express her feelings through a medium that she enjoyed: writing. Sonja produced some essays quite worthy of the Gothic horror fantasies of Edgar Allan Poe and Mary Shelley, an example of which is reproduced in the epilogue. Quite often, on reading her literature to me, Sonja would burst into gales of laughter and state that she would never do "any of this stuff."

There were many other literary rituals in which Sonja participated to contest her father's abuse. I asked her to write a copy of a "covenant" which she believed best represented the contract that her father had forced upon her when she was a child. Toward the end of Sonja's therapy, she told me that she had rewritten the covenant as an adult. Sonja burned the original covenant and scattered the ashes to sea. The second document is now framed and hanging on Sonja's wall.

Therapy concluded after a further year during which Sonja continued to change her dress much more freely according to her fancy, rather than her need to maintain distance. Sonja had also entered a relationship with Les, a thirty-five-year-old computer analyst, who appeared to listen to her and respect her needs.

At our final session, Sonja gave me a planter filled with linaria, candytuft, and snapdragons, accompanied by the following letter:

> Dear Dr. Gunzburg,
> I'd like to say thank-you for all the help and love you have given me.
> I hope you have lots of good patients and lots of good jokes in the future.
> Thank you, Good-bye
>   Love Sonja xox.

Eighteen months later, Sonja came for a session to discuss the ending of her relationship with Les. They had decided that they were now traveling separate paths and had agreed mutually to part. Sonja expressed her sadness and grief but knives were no longer a cutting issue![2]

---

2. A shortened version of this story was originally published in *General Practitioner*, Vol. 1, No. 13, pp. 17–18. All names in this story have been changed to maintain confidentiality.

Epilogue: Sonja's Gothic Horror Fantasy

Creeping up the stairs, lightly on my tiptoes, in the dead of night, I had the carving knife in my hand, ready to murder Dad. I was excited and yet trembling. I also felt like I was choking. There were curtains on the windows letting in the light. All was quiet. All I could hear were the night sounds. Everything was still peaceful. I carefully opened their bedroom door and crept in. I stood over them while they were sleeping. I remember when I was a girl, I had a dream where someone was standing over me, but I couldn't see their face. Someone was threatening me and now I was doing it back to them. I wanted to kill them and I felt creepy and wildly excited. I could knife both of them and finally get my revenge.

I was clutching the carving knife—the type chefs used, with a black handle and a very nasty blade—in my right hand. Dad woke up as he sensed someone was there and I surprised him. He saw me and put his hand up to his forehead and tried to scramble away up the pillow, backing into the wall. I wasn't going to let him get away this time. I'd let him escape before, when he caused my breakdown by walking out on me and slinging me into *chaos, into* that black hole where my whole world had been pulled from under my feet and any sense of control and security I had had been carelessly thrown out the window as something *unimportant*. He was scared of me, as I now had the power, and I was going to taunt him with it and make him pay for all the confusion he had caused me. I could see that he was scared and I saw fear on his face. He was going to experience fear and the unknown, and the sexual control he had over me that was enough to send me into a feeling of rage-chaos, as I had experienced when I was little. I raised my hand and plunged my knife into his heart, repeatedly stabbing him, saying: "'There, that's for you!" and "You bastard!" I was smiling to myself and felt madly out of control.

Working myself up into a mad frenzy (like an orgasm), I ripped his chest open like a savage dog after it has killed its prey and his heart away from his body with my bare hands. I threw it to the ground like a possessed witch and laughed madly. I grabbed his two arms and ripped them out of their sockets. Being caught up in the excitement of the kill, I continued to hack his body up.

Mum was hysterical, her hands were up to her face, screaming. I spun around, screaming at her to shut up and threw my knife at her, straight into the middle of her throat. Her knees gave way and she fell to the floor. I chopped her up like a butcher when he is at the chopping block. I got a garbage bag from the kitchen and put their dismembered bodies into the bag and carried it downstairs like Santa carries his sack of toys over his shoulder. I threw them into the boot of the car and drove to Portsea's back beach. I walked a little way into the bush and dug a shallow grave and dumped their remains there.

As I killed Dad, I experienced the ultimate orgasm, which I had been saving for him. I will never have another one so good. All my emotions of love and hate had flowed down that knife handle onto the blade and into Dad.

He did not have a heart.

I felt drained. There was nothing left

I felt?? . . . what is it when a religious person purifies you???

What Doesn't Meet the Eye

Hava Tabenkin
Jezrael Valley, Israel

Four years ago on a cold December morning. . .

"The Cohen family is here again," I say to myself as I enter the clinic. "Whose turn is it today?" I ask myself somewhat wearily. Is it six-year-old Ron, two-year-old Nurit, or ten-year-old Tal? Sarah and Abraham, the parents, bring their three children to see me quite often for a variety of complaints and many times I wonder why they come at all. Ron is ill most often.

This time it is Ron. He has had a high temperature for a week and has been generally feeling quite poorly. His record shows that he has been seen three times this year with tonsillitis and received antibiotics after throat swabs grew streptococci. The examination today raises the possibility of infectious mononucleosis ("kissing disease"), and I find myself ordering a lot of blood tests. Again I ask the worried parents whether there are other problems in the family or at school. This time the mother tells me that Ron can't concentrate and that he doesn't function well either in first grade or at home with the family. She relates to me her difficulties with him in terms of discipline and overstepping limits. She reports that the child is seeing a psychologist and she hopes the situation will improve. In an authoritative and certain tone I explain the connection between psychosocial problems and physical illnesses, especially infections. I reassure them that, in my opinion, the present illness will soon pass. They leave seeming satisfied.

The blood tests come back confirming my suspicion of infectious mononucleosis. A few weeks later I get a report from the parents that, although the course of the illness was longer than expected, the child got better in the end. As I write my clinic note, I think about Ron briefly. He is a very bright boy, but I have always found his behavior to be a bit odd. In addition, he always looks so miserable. His mother, Sarah, is also a strange woman, with quirky mannerisms and a history of bulimia, which I'm not certain is completely resolved. I always wonder how she raises her children. I assert that Ron's behavior is similar to that of his unusual mother. I don't look into the matter too deeply and relate the frequent illnesses to disturbances in personal and family functioning, which I hope will resolve in time. I feel reassured that Ron is in therapy.

After the bout with infectious mononucleosis, Ron continues to visit me with recurrent episodes of fever for at least two more years. Unfortunately,

121

the communication with the psychological service is poor and I receive no progress reports on his treatment. During these two years another family, the Levis, also come to see me repeatedly—mainly Danny, aged twelve and a half, with breathing problems and cough. Asthma was diagnosed in the emergency room of the local hospital on one of the occasions he was taken there. Every time the complaints are similar: cough and difficulty breathing, which sometimes keep him awake at night. He misses many days from school. Although I never hear wheezing when examining his lungs and never witness any respiratory distress, I never succeed in uncovering any information which could have pointed to a different reason for his complaints, so I accept the diagnosis of asthma.

When Danny isn't treated by me, his parents take him to the hospital, where he receives all the latest medications by inhalation and injection. On his return from the hospital his mother invariably meets me with remarks such as: "You see! You missed it again." Despite this, I have tried my luck and asked her what she thought could possibly cause these attacks. "Everything is fine," she always claims. I feel I have no choice but to join the game and treat him every time as a simple case of asthma. Severe attacks occur when the mother is pregnant and the family is expecting a baby. I am satisfied—I am "right" after all; in one of the conversations I try, gently, to relate the attacks to Danny's fear of losing his status as the youngest child. I explain, most knowingly, that the baby represents a threat to him, and go on to explain the biopsychosocial model to the mother, the nurses, and anyone else who is prepared to listen. When Danny is about fourteen the attacks suddenly stop. I don't have an explanation for this, but I have often seen children show marked improvement in their asthma.

One day, about half a year ago. . . .

The phone rings and at the other end of the line I hear the anxious voice of our social worker, who asks for an urgent meeting. The same day we meet and she tells me the following astonishing story. One day this week Ron came home, burst into tears, and confessed to his parents that for over two years (up until six months previously), Danny had been abusing him sexually. Ron is now eight and Danny nearly fifteen. Danny was going to be appointed group leader of Ron's group and he was terrified that the abuse would start again. The frightened parents turned to the welfare services and the social worker and they invited Danny and his parents to a meeting. Danny was asked to tell his side of the story. "Well, there was something . . . ," Danny admitted, trying to downplay what he had done. He claimed that there were times when he asked Ron to undress and only "played" with him while they were both naked; and anyway, "Ron didn't object." The extent of the abuse was not clear (either then or now), and it was not clear if there was any penetration.

A short time after the social worker contacted me, a special committee of the local branch of the Ministry of Social Welfare discusses the case in consultation with police investigators. It is decided not to file a complaint with the police, but rather to demand that Danny start psychological treatment with a specialist in child abuse. Ron's parents, anxious that the whole kibbutz would find out about the incident, refuse to file a complaint with the police. They are also concerned that someone might hurt or insult their son. Although Ron is the victim, the anger about the exposure of the case might turn against him and his family.

No one can imagine my frustration and feeling of failure. How did the possibility of sexual abuse (or even just bullying) never cross my mind? Not only had I read about this extensively, but I had been told of Ron's behavior problems at home and at school. How could I go on treating recurrent infections and asthma, when such frightening abuse was going on under my very nose and no one was aware of it? How could it happen that the psychologist, whom Ron met every week for more than a year, did not establish a relationship of trust that would enable him to tell her the truth about what really troubled him?

I was now faced with more challenges. What should be the extent of my involvement as the family doctor? To what extent should I maintain neutrality? I had more questions than answers. I decided to have regular meetings with Ron's parents and try to support them. I also had a few meetings with Danny's parents but was unable to make any progress. I was shocked to discover that Danny's mother did not think his actions were so terrible. She was angry with Ron for consenting! What rationalizations! My contact with Danny stopped. He seemed ashamed to meet me, probably because he knew that I knew what had happened and felt uncomfortable. Maybe this points to feelings of guilt. I do hope that these feelings exist in him, since this may be the first step in the healing process.

Epilogue

We always thought that sexual abuse would not occur on a kibbutz, especially not between children. The welfare of the individual is part of kibbutz ideology, and there is high awareness of social problems. Education is also oriented toward mutual assistance. How wrong we were to think it would never happen here.

I was not happy with the decision to try to keep reports of the abuse quiet. In my opinion, a complaint ought to have been filed with the police, and the community should have been made aware. I believe that Danny, the abuser, has to be punished—otherwise how will he know his deeds were wrong? How will Ron recognize that what was done to him was immoral if the perpetrator is not punished? His self-esteem is already low; how can it be built up? It is not clear to me how much the "psychological help" is actually helping.

References

Antao, V., A. Maddocks, E. Street, and J. R. Sibert. 1996. A case-control study of somatic and behavioural symptoms in sexually abused boys. *Archives of Diseases of Childhood* 75(3):237–38

Buist, A. 1995. Childhood sexual abuse and adult psychopathology: relevance to general practice. *Australian Family Physician* 24(7):1229–31.

Cohen, S., E. De Vos, E. Newberger. 1997. Barriers to physician in treatment of family violence: lessons from five communities. *Academic Medicine* 72(1):519–25. (suppl.)

Herbert, C. P. 1991. Family violence and family physicians: opportunity and obligation. *Canadian Family Physician* 37:385–90.

Kirkengen, A. L., B. Schei, and S. Steine. 1993. Indicators of childhood abuse in gynecologycal patients in a general practice. *Scandinavian Journal of Primary Health Care* 11(4):276–80.

Mammen, G., and B. Olsen. 1996. Adult survivors of sexual abuse: do I have them in my practice? *Australian Family Physician* 254:518–24.

Mazza, D., L. Dennerstein, and V. Ryan. 1996. Physical, sexual and emotional violence against women: a general practice–based prevalence study. *Medical Journal of Australia* 164(1):14–17.

McCann, I. L., and L. A. Pearlman. 1990. Vicarious traumatization: a contextual model for understanding the effects of trauma on helpers. *Journal of Traumatic Stress* 3:131–49.

Rosenberg, M. L., M. A. Fenley, D. Johnson, L. Short. 1997. Bridging prevention and practice: public health and family violence. *Academic Medicine* 72(1): 13–18. (suppl.)

Tudiver, F., and J. A. Permaul-Woods. 1996. Physicians, perceptions of and approaches to woman abuse: Does certification in family medicine make a difference? *Canadian Family Physician* 42:1475–80.

Suicide

Reflections

Shimon Glick, Shmuel Reis, and Jeffrey M. Borkan

The inclination toward life or toward death is often decided by an instantaneous or, if you will, an impulsive tipping of the balance in one direction or another. A smile, a touch, a ray of sunshine may prevent suicide; a frown, a rejection, a pessimistic news item—a cloud—may tip the scales in the other direction. In other instances, the decision to end one's existence is the result of a lifetime of suffering or an uncontrolled drive resulting from mental illness.

The Talmud aptly compares a dying patient to a flickering candle, so fragile, so easy to extinguish. But in reality this analogy is valid about all of our existences. Just a hairbreadth separates life from death. Once the Rubicon has been crossed, once the soul has departed, there is no way back. Each of the four stories in this chapter projects a clear common message: the utter loneliness, real or imagined, of the individual contemplating suicide, and the redeeming power of having someone or something with whom to share one's life. That someone could be a divinity, as in the first story, in which Mr. Wilcox felt that he had been saved by heavenly intervention. In the third narrative, one physician who fortunately possessed the qualities of caring and initiative effectively reached out and responded in kind to Cyberspace Sam. In "The Hand of Life," just the touch sufficed. Tragically, the woman in Dr. Arnold's account had been grasping for some attention and warmth all her life, but no one in her community would respond. Instead, the community where she resided (we hesitate to call it her community) conspired, some members actively, others passively, to exploit her for their needs. The result, no less bizarre and tragic than her entire life, was the almost inevitable outcome of her total emotional isolation.

The rising incidence of suicide in recent years has captured the concern of health professionals and social scientists seeking to understand the phenomenon (Woodbury, Manton, and Blazer 1998; Arensman et al. 1995). Primary care practitioners feel a personal loss when a patient commits suicide. The nature of general and family practice is such that many suicidal patients have visited their physicians in the months before the attempt (Gorman and Masterton 1990). Some feel guilt at not identifying and preventing self-harm and even more when suicide is part of associated familial or random violence. One of the commentators (SR) can personally testify to the devastating effect on a provider's morale when a patient killed his two young children and then committed suicide after his call for help was not recognized during a clinic visit a few weeks earlier.

Literature on identifying patients at risk, better detection of depression [half of the suicidal patients are said to be depressed (Isacsson et al. 1994)], and the question of suicide prevention in primary care is abundant. Nevertheless, it is inconclusive (Feightner and Worral 1990; Appleby et al. 1996; Olfson et al. 1996). Patients in general practitioners' offices usually do not share with their provider their suicidal intent. Many simple questionnaires to detect depression (Froom and Hermoni 1993) and attempts to heighten clinical awareness and improved communication and psychosocial concern have been devised. Strategies for follow-up and shared care with mental health practitioners have also been suggested (Adam et al. 1983; Brown and Mengel 1990). However, the adoption of these efforts has been limited at best.

Suicide comes in many shapes and forms. The last few years have witnessed a number of instances of mass suicides, apparently on the advice of a charismatic cult leader. Most of the lives lost in these almost incomprehensible tragedies have been young, and often talented, healthy individuals. Another genre of suicide endemic to the Middle and Far East has been the fanatic fundamentalist suicide bomber, who feels confident of instant admission to heaven in return for his or her sacrifice.

People are particularly prone to suicide at specific periods of life. For example, teenagers, all too often in the turbulence of their life stage, may succumb to what seem to them to be insurmountable problems. And the elderly, facing the seemingly grim prospects of a life's closure that promises to be bleak and uncontrollable, may attempt suicide before their dignity is eroded.

In almost all of these situations the phenomenon has its unique epidemiology and natural history. All too frequently the media report a succession of suicides under similar circumstances, suggesting that hearing about another's suicide may tip the balance for the wavering individual. One such case involved an elderly, relatively healthy kibbutz couple, who committed suicide in Israel several years ago because they did not want to become an economic and social burden on their kibbutz. This suicide received considerable media coverage, much of it favorable. The family physician on the kibbutz subsequently told one of the commentators (SG) that several other retired individuals on the kibbutz related that they had been pressured by this event into feeling somewhat guilty at continuing to live. This kind of response, the occasional series of teenage suicides, and the cult mass suicides emphasize the societal consequences of even an isolated suicide. Even the staunchest advocates of individual autonomy cannot afford to ignore the impact their suicide has on others—well beyond one's immediate family and friends.

The most difficult dilemmas may be faced by individuals with terminal or chronic illnesses after failure of skilled professional efforts to relieve their physical and emotional suffering. These are the hard cases presented so poignantly by the advocates of physician-assisted suicide. Timothy Quill's (1991) eloquent description of his young leukemic patient, Diane, and other similar cases, argue forcefully for physicians to be permitted to assist such patients to end their lives mercifully. The subject remains contentious, however. The potential abuses of the aged, the disadvantaged, and the minorities, in an era of "bottom-line" managed care (Sulmasy 1995), are enormous. Even in the Netherlands, with a relatively high incidence of euthanasia, there is a question of serious ethical deterioration over the years (Gomez 1991).

The French sociologist Émile Durkheim (1952) believed that in earlier societies the individual was somehow shielded or protected from committing suicide by a sense of belonging to a group, be it family, religious, or other. This protective factor of the group is often accentuated during times of societal crises such as war, when suicide rates fall paradoxically. Masterton and Mander (1990) described a unique example of collective spirit by the reduction in emergency psychiatric admissions during and after the World Cup soccer finals. They postulated that individuals swept up in the common rooting for their team assumed a feeling of belonging and thereby were protected against suicidal inclinations.

The positive potential of a common cause contrasts with the deleterious effect of the feelings of isolation that characterizes terminal illness. These feelings of utter isolation from even one's closest family members are described most poignantly and brilliantly in Tolstoy's insightful masterpiece *The Death of Ivan Ilyich*. The isolation and feeling of total worthlessness is a potent stimulus to suicide. When these feelings are reinforced by society and family through the presentation of suicide as an acceptable, and even desirable alternative, tragic consequences may ensue (Hendin 1995).

What are our roles as family and general physicians regarding this topic? Each of the four physicians in this chapter attempted to intervene to save the life of the sufferer or, if that was not possible, to understand the circumstances that led to the suicide. Beyond this direct and obvious role, we believe physicians should be proactive in their communities to identify those at risk for suicide and to minimize the feelings of isolation and anomie which may lead individuals to end their lives. It behooves us as a civilized society to convey the message to every member of our communities that we care, that no person is alone, that anyone's death diminishes us all.

Finally, it should be remembered that physicians are themselves at risk of suicide. Stress, marital discord, burnout, access to potentially lethal substances—all play their role (Olkinoura et al. 1990; Rennert et al. 1990). Rates of anxiety, depression, and even lack of stable primary care are more prevalent among physicians than among the general public. The stories in this chapter do not reflect on this tendency, but no doubt, throughout this book, the burden of doctoring is clear.

Felo-de-se

Robin Hull
Warwick, United Kingdom

Mr. Wilcox entered the examining room as he always did. He looked the same, spoke in his usual hesitant disjointed fashion, and again asked for his repeat prescription. He then announced: "I think I'm going to tell you something you haven't heard before."

The doctor glanced from the speaker to the student sitting beside him and looked dubious. After a few years in practice it is unusual to hear anything new, but at least this should be interesting for the student. As the old man sat down the doctor mentally rehearsed an introductory history for the student: Herbert Wilcox, a moderately successful, retired bank manager, sixty-nine years of age and married (poor fellow) to a nagging, hypochondriacal wife who disparaged everything he did. Despite this continual source of stress in his life, Herbert had remained well until a few years ago, when he suddenly developed mild cardiac failure,[1] secondary to coronary artery disease,[2] which was now successfully controlled by medication. He had had a cancer of the large bowel resected successfully two years ago, and he was doing very well despite the stress at home.

"Yes?" prompted the doctor, avoiding any intonation which suggested that he was thinking, "*Now* surprise me."

"It happened about a week ago . . . yes it was just after that upset in Parliament. . . . I'd been reading the newspaper . . . the usual bad news about everything. . . . and I felt a bit low. I took my wife's breakfast tray up. . . . I'd spilt a bit of tea in the saucer . . . she gets upset easily and doesn't like things like that. Anyway I washed it up and took her another . . . it doesn't matter really. Then I sat and thought . . . there only seemed one thing to do. We've got a two-bar electric fire—it's quite a good one with a long flex. I plugged it in outside the bathroom and took all my clothes off. I filled the bath and got in holding the fire about chest height. . . . Then I dropped it."

"What happened?"

Wilcox seemed to wake up as if from a trance, gathered himself, and continued. "It took ages to drop. . . . Then it sputtered and fizzed and just went out."

Doctor and student lost their ennui in an instant, but they were silent,

1. Cardiac failure is inadequate pumping by the heart, usually producing an accumulation of fluids (in the lungs or ankles, for example).
2. Coronary artery disease (CAD) is an occlusion of the heart (coronary) arteries by aggregates of fat and blood cell products, which causes heart disease.

transfixed by the picture the old man conjured up. The picture was framed by the realization that the agony was barely concealed in the matter-of-fact manner and hesitating voice. Both wondered how so foolproof a method of self-destruction could have failed. The doctor, recovering, said, "You really meant to kill, didn't you?"

"Oh yes. I don't know why it didn't work. . . . I asked an electrician what would happen if you did that. . . . He just laughed and said it would be instant death." Again Herbert paused and studied the middle-aged doctor and enthusiastic young student for a moment before adding slowly, as tears formed in his eyes: "You know, I'm not a religious man but . . . well, it seemed something stopped it . . . it was not meant to happen." As he spoke, the unheeded tears overflowed to splash on his waistcoat. The doctor, covering his own astonishment, launched into the routine of mental history taking. Yes, the patient had been depressed, but seemingly only by world affairs. There was no apparent personal cause for opting out of life. He had deliberately chosen to kill himself by a method which he had thought could not fail. Now he felt much better and had no wish to end his life at all but in his rather vague way "wondered if some pills might be a good idea" in case he ever felt that way again.

He had been right. We had not heard that story before, nor were we likely to hear its like again. Detailed questioning produced a little more information. There was a two-day history of poor appetite, drinking a little more gin than usual, a great tiredness, and a depression, more crushing than he at first admitted. This combination made death a consummation devoutly to be wished, resulting in an impulse which would not have failed without what he clearly regarded as some sort of divine intervention. If he had succeeded, one can picture the horror of the wife's discovery, the summons to the doctor, and his difficult task of consoling the widow while explaining to her the course the law must take and the need to inform the coroner. And then the doctor would leave, after doing what was possible to console her, and ponder what could have passed through a man's mind in those last seconds before the flash of convulsive death. Here sitting in front of them was a man telling just that story.

Attempted suicide is a common emergency in general practice, but fortunately only a few cases result in a "successful death." Nevertheless, every doctor has experiences of self-poisoning, of terrible self-inflicted shotgun injuries, of drownings and hangings. All these leave their scars, always with the nagging question, could the problem have been foreseen and prevented by timely intervention? Here, the doctor and student were confronted by failure of method so incredible that they felt as though death had already happened and they were involved in both prevention and aftermath. But for now, what to do about poor Herbert Wilcox? To gain time for thought he was examined, but all proved normal. At the student's suggestion simple blood tests were carried out to monitor his digoxin and diuretics.[3] Meanwhile, doctor and student debated what to do. When asked, Herbert was emphatic that he did not want to see a psychiatrist. For a moment the option of coercion was considered: should this man, who admitted having been a danger to himself, be admitted to hospital under order? But then who would cope with Mrs. Wilcox? In any case, such action seemed a terrible invasion of an old man's life, especially since he now felt that the matter was behind him. There was something about his conviction of divine intervention which impressed one that he would not make another attempt to kill himself. The doctor smiled ruefully to himself when he thought what an inquest jury might say to that.

General practice, it has been said, is a matter of tolerance of uncertainty. Here such uncertainty dangled like Damocles' sword. If the doctor decided that informal psychiatric help was impossible and compulsory admission was ethically wrong, the only possible option was the uncertainty of letting the patient go home. He tried to safeguard himself, most importantly with a frank discussion of the whole affair. He also urged Herbert to return to see him after a day or two to get his blood test results, and the resolving depression was treated with a small dose of amitriptyline,[4] which might need adjustment. Last, Herbert was given an envelope marked "To be opened only in severe emergency." Inside on a sheet of notepaper were instructions to telephone a given number and to read to the answering doctor the signed message: "This man needs immediate help."

So Mr. Wilcox left the surgery, and doctor and student went home thoughtfully to a very late supper hoping that all would be well.

Herbert Wilcox lived for several more years before, ironically, developing pneumonia at his wife's funeral.

Epilogue

When discussing the case with a psychiatrist some time later the doctor was criticized for taking such a risk. The psychiatrist held that more restraint should have been used, arguing that in such a case where one violent action had occurred there might well be another and that the second might well be directed at Mrs. Wilcox.

What would you have done?

3. Digoxin and diuretics are drugs that control heart failure.
4. Amitriptyline is an antidepressant medication.

Going Round in the Wind

Csaba Arnold
Budapest, Hungary

Once upon a time. . . .

The early spring morning was cold, windy, and gleaming. The naked branches were moving slightly, drawing on the white walls of the homes in the village, while we were leaving it. Outside the houses, the overripe smell of the ground after the snow struck me. I was sitting on a hundred-year-old bike behind the policeman of the village, who was trying to avoid the thin covering of ice over the potholes on the road. The curious smell reminded me of something which was astonishing, special, and familiar to me, but I could not recognize it at that very moment. Michaelmas daisy? Death? Hospital ward? Dissecting room? I was not sure, but the last had the closest resemblance. It reminded me of my university life, which had ended two years before.

At that time I was the only family physician in the village with more than three thousand inhabitants, who mostly lived within a six-kilometer radius. The houses were built sixty to seventy years earlier, with the arrival of the immigrants—descendants of an old semi-Hungarian tribe now living nearby. The immigrants settled here, lived separately among themselves, and married only inside the village. Traditions, fashions, habits, and standards remained unchanged, reflected in the way of thinking and problem solving as well.

The policeman was taking me on his bike, riding as slowly and carefully as he could. Unfortunately, he was not too successful, and I felt as if I could fall off at any moment. Jolting and slipping from one hole to another, one of my arms was around the policeman's hip, the other was holding my doctor's bag. With the weaving of the bike I was moving from one side to the other. I was looking half-round, as if I was in front of an extremely wide screen observing a panorama of the landscape. The village was small. The farmhouses outside were scattered along the side roads like the jumps of chess knights. The unpaved side roads crossed the main road at each kilometer.

The intersection was covered with mud and water, running up and down the small "hills." Along the road there were no trees but from time to time a farmhouse appeared behind the flat ridge of the hills. The houses were small, as in fairy tales. They had bright white walls, small, black but glittering windows, dark gray roofs, and smoking chimneys. The houses were surrounded by leaf-lost trees, small farm buildings, and dogs running up and down; yelping at each other, the canines were clearly alarmed at the appearance of the bike, frightening us with the thought that they might break their chains.

Suddenly we left the main road and were slipping on the muddy ground of the side road. The first house which we were approaching seemed to be smaller than the others but looked like the older ones. Near the broken wood fence the bike was blocked and stopped as if we were hit by a big hand. The sight we faced was curious, surprising, but picturesque.

In the middle of the empty courtyard, a lone well was standing, fenced with dark, broken wood. The sight we witnessed shocked us. There was a woman hanging on the upper end of the crossbar sweep, on the long, black wood. She was suspended with her head tilted aside as if she were wondering. The bright sun was shining through the naked branches onto her body. She was swinging in the breeze, slowly turning from one side to the other. She had committed suicide. The scene was as absurd as a scene in an avant-garde film: the picture has nearly no meaning or is so deep that no ordinary person could understand.

It started about ten days earlier.

I first met the woman two Thursdays ago; it was a very busy day. That morning both the surgical suite and the waiting room were more crowded than ever before. There was a loud knock on the door to the surgery room, nearly breaking it. The two nurses and I all jumped to open it, thinking there was an urgent case. Opening the door wide we saw an excited woman standing there. She ran inside and began to yell, "I was raped last night!"

There was more to the meaning of her sentence. She stated she was not only raped, but deflowered as well. I was urged to investigate her immediately and to give an official report about what had happened. She wanted the young, twenty-three-year-old man to be charged and sentenced to prison. She kept shouting in a high, unnatural voice, repeating the same simple sentence. I tried to calm her down, so she might clarify what had happened.

In the first version, the previous night, a young man broke into her home through the safely closed door and raped her several times. As she repeated it the story became more detailed. I was surprised to hear that it had happened not only once, but continuously every night for weeks. Everything in her story got darker and more mysterious. How did it happen? Did the same person repeat the same rape every night? The whole story got more and more confusing and did not sound true. It was impossible to clarify whether there was a rape. Her voice became clear, sharp, and loud from time to time, and I was pressed by her and my oldest nurse to do something about it. The nurse was seventy, and had worked for forty years as a midwife. She knew all the inhabitants from birth.

To stop the quarrel, the woman was examined, but no signs of rape could be observed. My findings were that no rape or wound could be ascertained. I told her that there was nothing which confirmed her claim, and no evidence against the young man. The deflowering had happened many years before; she was now fifty-three.

She did not accept my opinion and loudly requested a specialist. I tried to change her mind, but it was all in vain. I wrote the referral letter and she went away appearing satisfied with the result. I rang up the gynecologist in the town hospital detailing the story and asked him to help find a peaceful solution. Soon I forgot all about it. It was a busy day with more serious cases.

Now the policeman and I stood there, petrified.

Some old farmers, women, and even some children had gathered around us, turning to us expectantly for an explanation. The answer was already on their faces, however. She was dead. The policeman lifted the body and cut the rope, laying her gently on the ground. I made a formal investigation. It was a rather picturesque scene; the body on the ground by the well and the doctor on his knees. Supervising behind the doctor, the policeman, with a serious and official expression on his face with a sense of his importance. The others were standing around us like an ancient choir, watching and controlling what was happening. Not too far from the group a barking dog was sitting with his head and tail down and his face sad and dark. The silence was interrupted only by the policeman's voice: "Stupid woman, how stupid she was."

The wind was blowing, moving the branches and the lonely rope. My mind was empty; I could not understand the death or the cause of the suicide. It all seemed unbelievable to me. This was stupid, I agreed.

We returned to the surgery office where we were greeted by the nurses, full of questions. Was she really dead? Was it a suicide? When and how did it happen? The two nurses competed with each other, firing their questions at us at a rapid rate. Before we could even answer, they would formulate what they thought was the best answer. They discussed with the policeman what they already knew, adding more and more information. Somehow, the picture got clearer.

Prologue

The story began when the ugly girl became a middle-aged woman. After her parents died, she did not want to be alone, but nobody was around for her to marry. The loneliness intensified, and then from the neighborhood the first young man came. His visits were for one reason, which was duplicated by others in the area for weeks on end. A young man would visit her home in the night, say what he wanted, and get it. There was no rape involved, as all acts were consensual. Intercourse occurred on several occasions with several men, with no other involvement. They were together for the nights with no real feelings, no communication, and no promises. The young men always went away and disappeared as a dream, if she had any dreams at all. From the surrounding farms the young men appeared out of the dark fog and disappeared back into it. The contacts lasted for a short time and rarely longer than a few days. But she was not alone any more. Everybody knew everything in the neighborhood, and the wind blew the message far. Here was a woman, ugly but willing to teach the boys of physical love. Everyone felt she was the teacher except for her. She thought of these acts as the medicine against her loneliness. Her loneliness appeared to be solved, but only for some hours or days. She began to view this as a normal part of her life. She represented the "bad" when spoken of to the farmers' daughters, but she was a necessity and habit, a part of everyday life.

She felt old. She felt each young man that came to visit would be the last. Finally, one man came to her and the attachment became different. She wanted to possess him, like everything else she had around her in the farmyard. Not only his body, but the person, the soul, and the permanent presence were desired. This contact lasted longer than the others. They met and were in contact for three or four months. In her state of mind, it was a real "marriage." Suddenly, the man said he wanted to stop and after the last night he did not come again.

She was frightened that he might be the last man in her life. In her simple mind the solution was to go to the doctor and claim something that would force him to come back. In a normal family the father or the brothers were sent to the "fiancee" to make him marry her. In this case I was the one who could have helped, and I did not do it. She went to another physician, a specialist, but he too did nothing. She lost all hope and escaped into death.

Epilogue

My formalities were over and she was left lying on the ground. The official procedure began; they waited for the coroner and the detectives. The policeman transported me back on the old bike. The sunshine seemed colorless and the shadows were growing as if the nature had been mourning. I was in shock, and the road and the panorama did not interest me. Eventually we arrived back at the village. The houses were the same; white, striped by the shadows of the trees and branches. I was a young physician, and each case of death depressed me. Deep in my heart something told me I was responsible, and I had not done the best. I could not determine where I went wrong and how it could have been prevented. The houses and the trees did not answer me.

Time to time this "film" runs through my mind: I see myself looking at the village, the farmhouses, the bad road, the old bike, the small farmhouse, and the woman on the rope swaying with the wind. The picture was a curiosity of my youth. Envisioning it makes me young again, as I too am going round in the wind.

Slowly I forgot her; I did not want to think of it. Four years later I moved to another practice and began to teach students at the local university. I regularly spoke of the responsibility of the physician and the mistakes that can occur in family practice. More important, I spoke of how a physician, myself in particular, could live with them. Some cases were reported, and her story came to my mind. When I first told her story, I spoke only of the situation and the scene. The class, however, questioned the causes and I was forced to analyze it in its complexity. In retrospect, I understand that her first visit was a cry for help, but I did not realize it at the time. As I grew as a physician, I learned more about suicide and how to recognize and avoid a life-threatening situation. In teaching the circumstances of her death, the importance of noticing signs of despair and depression were ingrained into my practice. It is something I will not forget.

Cyber-Family Practice: A Story in Three Parts

Robert C. Like
New Brunswick, New Jersey

A "Clinical Encounter" on the Internet

It is approximately five o'clock on a hot July afternoon. I have just returned to my medical school office after a busy and tiring day seeing patients at our Family Practice Center. I check my phone messages, mail, and calendar. A host of academic tasks await me—committee meetings, student advising, lectures to the residents and medical students, a letter of recommendation that needs to be written, a journal manuscript to review. Multiple competing obligations comprise the life of an academic family physician. Fortunately there are no emergencies, and it looks as if I will be able to go home a little earlier tonight.

It occurs to me that I last checked my E-mail about a week ago. I am still fairly new to the Internet and do not yet make routine use of the information highway for communication purposes. Eventually I may become more comfortable with cyberspace. "How wonderful it is to be connected to people throughout the world," I muse to myself. I turn on my computer, get into my electronic mailbox, and discover the following three-day-old E-mail message:

Hello! Was just snooping around the hostname files on my server and came across "rwja.umdnj.edu" and "njmsa.umdnj.edu" so I thought I would see if I could find your user id. Now you have my address, as well as my web page address.

Actually, while I'm here I hate to bother you with a professional question, but at least this way you can answer when you have the chance. I've been on and off depressed (more on than off for several years now). I first saw a psychotherapist several years ago during my freshman year of college, after finding myself spellchecking a suicide note at three am [sic] one Saturday night. I felt better after several sessions with her, but my troubles were not over. As soon as something would go wrong, as soon as the stress would go up, the depression would return, along with thoughts of suicide. My mother knows about that first suicidal time, but not any of the others, and my dad doesn't know any more than [sic] I am periodically depressed. Psychotherapy seems to work only temporarily, which is why a friend of mine, who is on Prozac herself, suggested that maybe I needed something like Prozac or other antidepressant drugs to cure me of this before I do go too far one night. I was just curious as to how expensive such drugs are, what is involved in determining if I do indeed need anything like that and what is involved in obtaining whatever is necessary. I assume that since I first sought help three years ago, under a different insurance company/plan, that it would be labeled as "preexisting condition" and therefore not be covered. But if it's at all possible for me to do it, I think it's worth it. Not sure how to tell my parents, or even if I should, but I guess that's something to consider later on

Thank you for any help/information/advice you can give me.

Sam (pseudonym)

I sit back in my chair and sigh deeply. I know this person. His family comes to our Family Practice Center. What a dilemma. What do I do now?

Personal Introspection and the Auto-BATHE

It has been said that before acting, one should always "take one's own pulse" first. I take a deep breath and fortunately remember a helpful interviewing technique known as the BATHE,[5] which we teach our residents and medical students to use in caring for patients. Well, it's time to BATHE myself (i.e., perform an "Auto-BATHE"). I ask myself the following series of questions:

B. **Background:** What's going on?

Sam has reached out to me for help via E-mail. He is depressed and has gone for individual counseling in the past. He is concerned that he may have a more serious depression requiring medication. He has contemplated suicide in the past. He is also not sure whether or what to tell his family about his condition. He is looking for information, support, and professional guidance.

A. **Affect:** How do I feel about it?

I experience a mixture of emotions including surprise, shock, and dismay. My day was exhausting enough and the last thing I needed was a new and complex situation such as this to deal with. However, a person is in distress and a life is potentially at risk. This must take precedence.

T. **Trouble:** What troubles me the most?

I am worried, of course, about Sam's depression. How serious is the suicide threat? How can I best assess the situation in order to provide assistance? I also am concerned about the best way to interact with Sam and his family since we all live in the same community. What is the right thing to do clinically, ethically, and legally?

H. **Handle:** How should I handle the situation?

A variety of practical questions go through my mind. Do I need to deal with this situation now or can it wait till tomorrow? Should I send an E-mail response? Should I send a certified letter? Should I try to telephone Sam (presuming I can locate his phone number)? Should I speak with Sam's parents? Should I contact one of my psychiatric colleagues for advice? Does Sam have his own personal physician and if so, should I contact him or her? Does this E-mail com-

---

5. M. R. Stuart and J. A. Lieberman III. *The Fifteen Minute Hour: Applied Psychotherapy for the Primary Care Physician,* 2nd ed. (Westport: Praeger, 1993).

munication constitute a "clinical encounter?" Does this encounter need to be documented in the medical record, and if so, how? The questions go on and on.

E. **Empathy:** A little bit of self-empathy.

I force myself to stop thinking and try to give myself a "mental pat on the back." I will try the best I can and hope everything will work out. So much for a quiet night at home.

Patient- and Family-Centered Clinical Praxis

I decide that I will try first to locate Sam's phone number as his E-mail appears to have been sent from his college. I make a long-distance call to the campus operator only to learn that Sam is not registered there for this summer. No luck. I drive home and tell my wife that I have a "clinical emergency" that needs to be dealt with. She is a nurse and is understanding as always.

Sam's family lives in the community and perhaps I can find out where he is. I go over to his house and ring the bell. Much to my surprise and relief, Sam answers the door himself. He is at home with the rest of his family. As he is an adult and has sent me a confidential and personal communication, I invite him over to my home saying, "I received your E-mail. Would you like to come speak with me about the information you requested?" He agrees and his family do not seem to suspect that anything is wrong.

My wife needs to run some errands; she leaves me with our two-year-old son, who is happily playing with his trains. Sam and I sit in the living room. I thank him for his E-mail message and over the next fifteen minutes learn more about what has been going on in his life. We discuss the duration, frequency, and severity of his depressive symptoms, what he has told his family so far, and what types of help he has sought. Clinically, I conclude that he is not actively suicidal but does indeed have a *major* depressive disorder[6] which will require antidepressant medications. I discuss this with Sam and ask him if he would like to have a family meeting where we can share his E-mail communication and discuss potential treatment options with his parents. He agrees to this and internally I heave an inaudible sigh of relief. Sam goes home, and both he and his parents return fifteen minutes later. Over the next half hour, we discuss my clinical findings and treatment recommendations. I commend Sam for his courage and willingness to obtain help. His parents fortunately are very supportive and understanding, and a referral to a psychiatrist is accepted. Everyone smiles and shakes hands. The genie is out of the bottle.

After Sam and his family leave, I reflect further on what has transpired this evening. A powerful personal learning experience. A gratifying clinical en-

---

6. Major depression disorder is a state of dejection, melancholia, and unresponsiveness to surroundings in a severe form.

counter. A ratification of the family systems paradigm of health care.[7] I believe that all will work out for the best. I return to playing with my son and his trains. My wife comes home and asks how my day has been. . . .

Yes, the Internet is indeed a wondrous creation of technology and is enabling us to become an interconnected global community. As we increasingly travel on the many byways of the electronic information highway, I wonder what new challenges await us and what the impact will be on the doctor–patient relationship and the practice of medicine.

7.   Family systems paradigm is the notion that family relationships reciprocally influence health (both by coping with and by producing or protecting from ill-health).

The Hand of Life

Dov Steinmetz

Kibbutz Yagur, Western Galilee, Israel

As a practicing family physician on the kibbutz where I live, I had treated R. H. a number of times for arthritic pains. A lovely woman, aged eighty-two, she and her husband and family were all members of the kibbutz, but at this stage, I could not claim to really know her or her background. This was about to change.

One morning I was informed that R. H. had just been released from the hospital, after an attempted suicide. The incident had been handled medically, with attention paid only to the physical problems. Now it was to fall to me to pick up the pieces.

The request was for me to make a house call, as the attending family physician. In this capacity, I would be able to monitor the situation and take any steps I deemed necessary for follow-up. I duly made my way to the compact kibbutz apartment where R. H. lived.

I found myself in a darkened room. She was lying down and I carefully and quietly made my way to her bedside. I made my presence known to her, and gently shook her hand. Then, seated, I projected as much compassion and empathy as possible, while she lay there, heavy-eyed and heavy-hearted. She started speaking, very softly, barely above a whisper, and I strained to hear what she was telling me.

She had suffered a terrible loss four years previously. Her beloved daughter had tragically died from metastatic breast cancer, a loss to which she had, obviously, still not adjusted. It was painfully clear that they had enjoyed a particularly close relationship, and ever since her death, R. H. had, daily, been going to the cemetery, where she would have long conversations with her dear, departed daughter. Yet her anger was still quite undiminished, and she could not accept the untimely death of the much younger woman. She kept questioning the absurd situation, that she, a woman of eighty-two, should still enjoy such rude good health, when her daughter had died so young. She railed against the cruelty of a mother having to bury her child. While in this frame of mind, she had decided that she would painstakingly accumulate as many sleeping pills as it would take, and then she would take the tablets and so be united, at last, with her beloved daughter.

I felt myself very well prepared for this kind of encounter, as I had just returned from a year in the United States where I had studied the subject of the "Family Physician and the Dying Patient." I found myself uttering the "wise" things I thought needed to be said, and before I left her, I suggested that she pay me a visit at my office within the coming few days.

Some days passed before she turned up at my consulting rooms. However, this was a very different person. She was ebullient, almost euphoric, eager to tell me a story.

As a young child, at the tender age of six, she was living in Poland with her parents and extended family. Included in this extended family was a beloved and respected grandfather, who was a practicing Hasidic Jew. The little girl had two disabilities to deal with: not only did she stutter, but she also had another embarrassing problem—she suffered from enuresis (bedwetting). A heavy load for a little six-year-old to carry.

Her mother was afraid to send her to school in such a condition, so she took her to see a famous physician who came from Vienna once a month to the local hospital. The doctor examined her, spoke with her, and gave her some medication—all in vain. The problem continued, much to the concern of all involved. Her grandfather told her mother to take the child to the rabbi in a nearby city. He believed that the rabbi was the only one who could cure her. So the whole family traveled in a horse-drawn carriage for an entire day to the rabbi's house. She distinctly remembered that the rabbi had beautiful blue eyes, white skin, and a lovely long beard. He put his hands on her head and said: "Go home child, and with God's help you will be well." He gave her a good-luck charm to wear for a whole year. Sure enough, upon arriving home after this eventful visit to the rabbi, the little girl not only spoke perfectly normally, but she was no longer suffering from enuresis. From that day on, she felt that the rabbi had given her his blessing, and that she would be protected and safe for her whole life.

"I don't remember what you told me when you came to visit me last week," she said, "but I do remember your hands. When you shook my hand, I felt my rabbi again. You gave me the hand of life." She then continued: "I will never try to commit suicide again. As far as my beloved daughter, may her dear soul rest in peace. She will have to be patient and wait until my time comes. Then, and only then, will I join her."

References

Adam, K. S., J. Valentine, G. Scarr, and D. Streiner, 1983. Follow-up of attempted suicide in Christchurch. *Australia-New Zealand Journal of Psychiatry* 17(1):18–25.

Appleby, L., T. Amos, U. Doyle, B. Tomenson, and M. Woodman, 1996. General practitioners and young suicides: a preventive role for primary care. *British Journal of Psychiatry* 168(3):330–33.

Arensman, E., A. J. Kerkhof, M. W. Hengeveld, and J. D. Mulder, 1995. Medically treated suicide attempts: a four year monitoring study of the epidemiology in the Netherlands. *Journal of Epidemiology and Community Health* 49(3):285–89.

Brown, R. L., and M. B. Mengel, 1990. Physicians' role in managing emotionnally distressed patients already in psychotherapy. *Journal of Family Practice* 31(4):381–86; 386–8. (disc.)

Durkheim, É. 1952. *Suicide: A Study in Sociology.* London: Routledge and Kegan Paul.

Feightner, J. W., and G. Worral. 1990. Early detection of depression by primary care physicians. *Canadian Medical Association Journal* 142(11):1215–20.

Froom, J., and D. Hermoni. 1993. The inventory to diagnose depression (IDD) in primary care patients. *Family Practitioner* 10(3):312–16.

Gomez, C. F. 1991. *Regulating Death: Euthanasia and the Case of the Netherlands.* New York: Free Press.

Gorman, D., and G. Masterton. 1990. General Practice consultations patterns before and after intentional overdose : a matched control study. *British Journal of General Practice* 40(332):102–5.

Hendin, H. 1995. Selling death and dignity. *Hastings Center Report* 25:19–23.

Isacsson, G., P. Holmgren, D. Wasserman, and U. Bergman. 1994. Use of antidepressants among people committing suicide in Sweden. *British Medical Journal* 308(6927):506–9.

Masterton, G., and A. J. Mander. 1991. *Psychiatric emergencies: Scotland and the World Cup finals. British Journal of Psychiatry* 156:475–78.

Olfson, M., M. M. Weissman, A. C. Leon, D. V. Sheehan, and L. Farber. 1996. Suicidal ideation in primary care. *Journal of General and Internal Medicine* 11(8):447–53.

Olkinoura, M., S. Asp, J. Juntnen, K. Kattu, L. Strid, and M. Aarimaa. 1990. Stress symptoms, burnout and suicidal thoughts in Finnish physicians. *Social Psychiatry and Psychiatric Epidemiology* 25(2):81–86.

Quill, T. E. 1991. Death and dignity : a case of individualized decision making. *New England Journal of Medcine* 324:691–94.

Rennert, M., L. Hagoel, L. Epstein, and G. Shifroni. 1990. The care of family physicians and their families. *Family Practitioner* 7(2):96–99.

Sulmasy, D. P. 1995. Managed care and managed death. *Archives of Internal Medicine* 155:133–36.

Woodbury, M. A., M. G. Manton, and D. Blazer. 1988. Trends in US suicide mortality rates 1968 to 1982. *International Journal of Epidemiology* 17(2):356–62.

Death

Reflections

Kathy Cole-Kelly

What can prepare a physician for dealing with such a complex, universal and intimate topic as dying and death? For some, the initiation begins when a family member or friend dies. Readiness for the actual involvement may be furthered by participation in educational forums in which individuals discuss issues related to death and dying. Classes that debate issues of euthanasia, DNR (do not resuscitate) orders, and choices of pain management in the face of death can equip the physician with a greater intellectual familiarity. But perhaps nothing will prepare a physician better for dealing with the complex and arbitrary aspects of death and dying than personal and poignant professional experiences. That is the beauty of the stories in this chapter. They transport the reader into the tender reflections of physicians still wrestling with the breadth of challenges dealing with death and dying.

The stories here describe a range of experiences. Some of the stories are from the novice phase of the physician's practice and reveal the *dis-ease* the physician felt about caring for the dying patient. The dis-ease springs from multiple causes: inexperience, lingering guilt, and astonishment at the level of professional responsibility. Other stories reveal an important metamorphosis in understanding that leads to a greater ease of involvement in the dying process. Most frequently what facilitated a better doctor–patient–dying relationship was the physicians learning more about the patient either through a history with the patient or knowing the patient's family members.

The stories span the cultures of the United States, Scandinavia, South American, the United Kingdom, and Canada. They also span communities—from urban poor to rural poor. However, the difference in setting mainly offers a variety in landscape, from inner-city squalor to rural fields. Otherwise, the cultural and physical landscapes in each of these stories are more background than foreground. Although in cultural settings thousands of miles apart, thematic commonalities diminish geographical differences. The stories reveal the struggles, the rewards, and the enduring memories of the experience.

"Had I committed malpractice?" "Could I have done something else?"

"My first reaction was one of guilt"—these quotes from this chapter reveal the persistent guilt that often visits a physician whose patient is dying or has died. These are important concerns for physicians to wonder about with their patients. There seems to be an inevitability about guilt accompanying the physician. It isn't all bad. Guilt can have a constructive role in individual development by promoting review of and self-reflection on behavior. If the guilt is a passing, yet serious wonder, versus a paralyzing end point, it's a worthy emotion.

It is important for physicians to have access to some constructive process to work through insecurities. In "The Next Generation," the physician, after raising his self-doubts, found comfort when his colleague reassured him. Physicians often benefit by examining questions that arise after an unexpected death or an underanalyzed dying process. These poignant stories of death need listeners so that the physician can better understand the complexities of each situation. Whether the listeners be colleagues, partners or spouses, or a formal process such as a Balint group—a meeting of family physicians to discuss difficult doctor–patient relationships, particularly the physicians' contribution—(Balint 1952), the telling and wondering can provide a forum for assuaging the guilt and for gaining useful insights. Providing a forum for physicians in training and practice can be a useful way of encouraging them to seriously look at their work (Cassell 1985:210) It also teaches the trainees the value of processing the intensity of their feelings and of appreciating the common experience of guilt that comes when working with dying patients and grieving family members.

A natural companion to the feelings of guilt is the sense of enormous responsibility. "My every decision might be a life and death decision," writes Stanley Smith in "The Next Generation." This sense of responsibility comes through in each of the stories: responsibility for taking over someone else's patients while they are on vacation; responsibility for making decisions; responsibility for inheriting a colleague's entire practice; responsibility for being responsive to a patient's request to end life ("I rely on you to let me out if it gets too bad"); responsibility to a dying patient's spouse's request. With each of the tellers of these stories, one can feel the weightiness of these considerations, the seriousness of the responsibility.

One way of coping with the sense of responsibility is revealed in the stories in which the physician collaborates with the families—not in any way to shirk the professional responsibility of using one's knowledge and skills, but to recast the sense of who is in the circle of responsibility (McDaniel, Hepworth and Doherty 1995). The families are critical resources to both the doctor and the dying patient. The families often hold the key to unlock what otherwise are seen as strange or resistant positions or beliefs, fostering a more satisfying process of dealing with the dying through the relationship story. In each story, one or more family members were central considerations: in "The Promise," a wife could clarify her husband's desire to die at home;

in "Jaw Pain and Panic," a husband could help a physician hear the patient's pain; and in "Mr. Jones Needs to Be DNR'ed," the wife could be the resource for understanding why DNR had been mistakenly requested. In contrast to the individual vision of deteriorated patients, the family stories of vibrancy, vitality, and passionate relationships emerged. By gathering the family perspective and stories, the physician could have a wiser understanding of the patients' wishes regarding their last requests. Without those stories, the patients are more unidimensional: Angus was dying; Mr. Jones was refusing treatment. By understanding the patients, their relationships, and thus their beliefs, the physician can help in navigating the journey to death (McDaniel, Campbell, and Seaburn, 1993).

"Venancio's Legacy" presents a unique perspective: a doctor who had known the patient when the doctor was a mere child. This is a wonderful twist to the doctor knowing the patient over time. The power of this long-term important childhood friendship creates a rich text about connection and caring during the dying process. The warmth and attachment this physician feels for his friend, now dying patient, is set in vivid counterpoint to the colder, detached objective approach of the other physicians in the hospital. In this story, the history with a patient seems to make a monumental difference in the gentle nature with which the physician approaches death and dying.

Compare this to situations in which the physician did not have access to as many clues to the situation, where the physician, less familiar with the patient and the family context, was at times at a greater disadvantage. In "The Next Generation," the physician doesn't know what the mother's threshold for concern about her children is for gauging the seriousness of her call for help; in "The Farmer's Thumb," the physician is hearing only the farmer's perspective about his thumb and later his wish for dying rather than hearing his wife describe her sense of how he is changing or discover her feelings about his wish to die.

Home visits, a phenomenon seldom practiced in the United States but mentioned in several of these tales, clearly facilitate the gathering of important threads to the relationship story. Dr. Hull's home visit to Mr. Bradney leads to his greater understanding of the patient's presenting problem; Dr. Smith's visit to the Y family helps him see the baby in the context of the impoverished family; Dr. Feldman's visits to the Jacksons allows her to see the beauty of their relationship. None of these contextual pieces, which help put the dying in a context of care and community, would have been available without the home visit.

Finally, we learn in these stories the importance of rituals. We know that rituals for major life events are an important mechanism for paying tribute to the event, for acknowledging it in a "public" forum, whether that be in the baby's room doing the physical exam to confirm the death or, as in the statement "Angus is dead" to a roomful of family members who already know (Imber-Black, Roberts, and Whiting 1988). The doctor–patient relationship is full of rituals: the way the exam is conducted, the laying on of hands, the opening and closing of the visit. Every culture has rituals that give the members of that culture an identity. It is the absence of a ritual that can make one feel out of place, lonely, lost. What we didn't hear about in these stories were the rituals that the physicians participated in after the patients died. Did they go to the patient's funeral? Did they write a letter? Did they go to their spouses and talk? Did they say a prayer? Did they pause? Did they meet with their support group? Rituals have a role in offering comfort as well as acknowledging a major life event. They can help reduce guilt, acknowledge responsibility, connect one with a larger community of others who are suffering losses. It would be valuable to know the story of the rituals each of these physicians used to gain comfort. Storytelling can be a ritual that may help students and residents who will be confronting the enormity of life and death issues that physicians face (Cole-Kelly, 1994).

I am confident these stories will be comforting and informative to students and practitioners alike. The stories reveal the multiple ways that physicians relate to patients and their families confronting dying and death. The stories describe the ongoing reflections of these intimate relationships. The details of the relationship contexts distinguish these stories more than the cultural contexts.

Several of the authors write in their stories how they yearned for more discussion of death and dying during their training years. The art of talking with the dying patient, and the family, is undertaught in medical school and residency (Field and Cassell 1997). There might be one or two sessions on ethical dilemmas around euthanasia, DNR, or how to talk to a dying patient. But these discussions rarely include the challenges of being with patients who are dying, of caring for patients who are dying, of listening to their family members, and finally of coping with our own emotions. The stories in this section can be part of that teaching process. They so well articulate the major themes of physicians dealing with death: revealing the deep wells of guilt so often stirred up, the gnawing wonder about responsibility for patients, the importance of understanding the patient and family members' belief about the dying process, the demanding role for the physician when one is family-oriented, and finally, the thin line between the rational and the emotional response to dying and death.

The Next Generation

Stanley G. Smith
Saskatoon, Saskatchewan

The phone rang intrusively as I sat at my desk writing notes on the patient I had just seen. I picked it up.

"Dr. Smith?" A female voice.

"Yes," I said.

"Could you come out to the house and check the baby?" The voice had a dullness, an indifference, that a more experienced physician might have recognized as a warning sign. It was ten in the morning, I was running late, and four patients sat in my waiting room. It was my first week in practice, and it was a new experience to be solely responsible for the patient's care. I found it frightening to know, or at least to think, that my every decision might be a life and death issue. Making quick decisions was difficult; medical school and internship had not taught me how to handle simple nonmedical issues.

"What seems to be wrong?" I asked.

"The baby has diarrhea" Mrs. Y answered tersely.

"How bad is it? How many times a day ?"

"Oh, I don't know, he just seems sick. Are you coming out?" she asked.

"Yes," I said, "I'll be out as soon as I've finished seeing my patients in an hour or so."

"Okay," she said, gave me the address, and hung up.

It was one of those bright, hot prairie days, under a radiant blue sky. It was about two hours after the phone call as I drove northward through the city, into progressively seedier neighborhoods. I finally identified the house. It was a small wood frame house that had once been green. That much could be deduced from the occasional green chip of paint that still adhered to the wood. The small front yard was overgrown with weeds and strewn with garbage. The front door was slightly open and when I tried to ring the doorbell there was no sound. I could hear a baby crying inside the house. I tried rapping on the door with my knuckles, but still no response. I pushed the door open and walked inside.

The stench was unbelievable. The house was strewn with every type of litter imaginable: crusts of bread, paper, dirty clothes, unwashed dishes, toys, and garbage, in addition to dirt in every corner. I assumed the crying baby was my patient. I worked my way toward the kitchen and opened the door. Inside a four- or five-year-old boy had opened the refrigerator and seemed to be eating at random. He looked grubby, his face smeared with food, and a purulent discharge was running from his nose. A dirty little girl was trying to drag him over to the table to no avail.

A door opened and a fat, unkempt young woman with greasy-looking hair slouched into the room. "He's in there," Mrs. Y said, pointing to another room.

I felt anxious for a moment. I had expected to be directed toward the room where I had heard the crying. Even though I had visited slums before, and as a student completed many home deliveries in the slums of Dublin, I felt peculiarly uncomfortable. I walked into the room she pointed to, which was as grubby as the rest of the house. She pointed to a crib in the middle of the room. Under a pile of dirty covers lay a small body, white, with a sort of yellowish tinge to its waxy skin. The child was motionless, its limp form not much bigger than a ragged doll at the bottom of the crib. I pulled back the covers, horrified. Could the baby really be dead? Surely not in this day and age. How could this have happened? Was it my fault? Maybe if I had dropped everything and come to the house as soon as she phoned, I could have saved this little life.

Although the baby was obviously dead, I senselessly went through the ritual of performing a physical examination on the little body. Perhaps it was not senseless, for ritual does provide an opportunity to reflect on the present situation and give one an opportunity to collect one's thoughts.

"I'm very sorry to have to tell you the baby is dead," I said.

"Oh," she said, as though all this had nothing to do with her. "What do I do now?"

This was my first week in practice. Nobody in medical school had taught me what to do about anything like this. After all, medicine is all about saving lives and relieving pain and suffering, not disposing of dead babies. I knew enough to know that unexplained deaths had to be reported to the coroner. From the next room I heard the sister call to the small boy, "Get away from the fridge, Gary, you can't just keep taking food any time you want."

"I have to call the coroner," I said, embarrassed to have to mention such a thing. "I think there will have to be an autopsy, so you will have to bring him down to the hospital."

She didn't seem unduly perturbed, as though nothing had registered at all.

As I walked out of the house I glanced back. My last glimpse was of little Gary, being pulled away from the fridge by his sister, twin tracks of yellow-green snot running down his upper lip, delicately poised at the slightly upward incline, where the white skin met the pink.

Doctors have been trained to take a lot of responsibility, even for things they are not responsible for. As I drove back to the office that afternoon I felt, quite unrealistically, that perhaps, if I had only dropped everything and run straight out there, maybe I could have saved that baby. As I walked up to my office I stopped at the office of one of my senior colleagues, whom I had adopted as a mentor.

"What are you looking so grim about?" he asked me.

Jamie was a wiry, lean guy. He was kind, but with a short temper that went well with his clipped Canadian accent. He had been a fighter pilot in World War II, and somehow he looked it. He usually had a carton of cigarettes on his desk and a lit cigarette in his hand. When he had his heart attack a few years later, he got into his car, drove down to the emergency room, and walked in saying, "I'm having a heart attack, someone better do an EKG." He was right, he was having a heart attack.

"I just made a house call on a dead baby," I said. "If I had just run straight out when I got the call, maybe I could have got the kid into the hospital and we could have gotten some fluids into him and saved his life, but the mother didn't sound that concerned over the phone."

"How long was it between the phone call and the time you got out there?" he asked.

"A couple of hours," I said.

"Perfectly reasonable," he stated. "You know perfectly well there was nothing you could have done. You responded perfectly reasonably. Why don't I give the coroner a call on your behalf. I know the routine."

Although I never had a chance to repay Jamie for his kindness and support, I hope I have passed on the kindness and support he showed me to some of the young physicians I have worked with over the years. He called the coroner and put me in touch with the appropriate social services, who went out and visited the home. Not surprisingly, they decided the parents did not have the skills necessary to look after children. They were not deliberately cruel to the children; they merely lacked the capability to raise a child properly. The children were placed in a foster home, I was informed later. From time to time I thought of little Gary, who had no regular eating hours and would just forage through the fridge whenever he felt hungry. My thoughts turn to that last glimpse I had of him, with the snot running down his nose, and to his sister, not much older, looking after him.

Many years later, one of my duties was as medical officer for a high-security psychiatric prison. One morning, I was seeing patients regarding their general medical condition, when a polite young man came in to see me. He looked vaguely familiar. I picked up his chart and read his name. It was Gary Y. The same Gary Y I had last seen in that squalid house when I had attended his long-dead brother.

The Farmer's Thumb

Robin Hull
Warwick, United Kingdom

It happened over thirty years ago; the scar is tender yet.

I suppose it was a mark of trust that George, my senior partner, had left me in charge of the practice for the first time. During my first year in the practice, while he was away, he had always hired a locum[1] to "help" me look after the thirty-five hundred patients scattered thinly over fifty square miles of rural central England. But after a full year in the practice and with the confidence of youth I knew I could cope with the workload for two weeks despite, in the early 1960s, a heavy domiciliary obstetric burden.[2] However, that was before I met Mr. Bradney.

The trouble started on the very first day. It seemed that the whole practice population had decided to be ill and the appointment system was soon swamped with urgent "extras." They waited with countrymen's patience as the waiting room overflowed into the street outside. They were lovely people. In those days, unlike today, the doctor, even one as inexperienced as I, was treated with courtesy and respect. If he was running late, that was because he was sought after and indispensable rather than disorganized and inadequate, as he would be thought today. So I struggled with the massed sick and even quite enjoyed the challenge . . . until I came face-to-face with Mr. Bradney.

On this occasion Bradney arrived unannounced and strode through the crowded waiting room, ignoring the receptionist's protests, and erupted into my consulting room as I showed a patient out. Hasty reference to the notes my red-faced receptionist handed me led me to misread his name and address him as "Bradley." Most people, when their names are mistaken, simply correct the error; not so John Bradney, who made an issue of it as if I had deliberately slighted him. During this I realized I had met him once before; I had not cared for him then either. To make matters worse I remembered that he was a close personal friend of George, my absent partner, with whom he regularly played chess. George had looked after Mrs. Bradney, whose life had changed from that of an extremely active farmer's wife and mother of several tough farming sons to a wheelchair existence caused by multiple sclerosis. Perhaps, I pondered charitably during Bradney's angry reaction to my mispronunciation of his name, his outburst was due to the stress of looking after his crippled wife.

Bradney had come from the north of England and was a very hardworking, successful farmer; his tough life had made him intolerant of fools. He was

1. A locum is a physician hired for a short while to replace a GP on a vacation.
2. Domiciliary relates to delivery of babies in the home.

a man not given to hiding his irritation when things did not go smoothly. Despite this I remembered my partner's admiration of how he coped with his crippled wife. Bradney finally subsided into the chair by my desk, still huffing about my mistake with his name, demanding: "Where's George?" On learning that his usual doctor was away on holiday, he made it quite clear that he did not think much of "seeing the second team." However, he put up with me because the problem was nothing more than a "funny feeling" in his right thumb. Suppressing my irritation with this demanding, angry patient presenting with self-confessed trivia, I tried to extract more history. He kept reiterating "it's just this funny feeling in my thumb," managing to suggest by his tone that even the simplest doctor fresh from medical school should immediately recognize a diagnosis. With no other information, local examination was unhelpful. I reassured him that at the age of fifty-eight, this was unlikely to be anything but a little arthritis. I suggested aspirin and the farmer left only partially mollified.

Without further incident I forgot Mr. Bradney and his thumb, but not for long. Two days later he was back, aggressively insisting on more action. The thumb was, if anything, "funnier," but not to me. This time full examination was equally unrewarding and he seemed so angry that I again wondered at my partner's choice of friends. Perhaps he sensed this because he said he was busy with harvest and could not manage "with one bloody 'and." In desperation I prescribed stronger analgesia.

The next day Bradney was on the phone, abusing the receptionist and demanding an urgent visit. I was busy with a prenatal clinic and getting very tired of my partner's friend; I wondered how long I could remain civil with him. I refused his request for an urgent visit, which would mean leaving the clinic, but —controlling my own anger with some difficulty—I agreed to see him at home later.

When I arrived at the farm, across a partly cut cornfield, the combine harvester was parked by the house. I was seething inside but he had quieted and I found him lying on his bed looking puzzled. I remembered wise teaching that a doctor under stress should always make a careful examination, since there was nothing like a diagnosis missed by an angry doctor to cause one to appear a fool. I repeated history and full examination. These, as before, were quite unhelpful. I was about to deliver an extremely stern lecture when Bradney said: "Its 'appening again." In a second he had developed a full-blown Jacksonian fit.[3]

The picture suddenly focused. A trivial, unexplained symptom presented by a farmer at his busiest time of year must indicate something more serious than I had realized. His emotional and unexpected outbursts, representing sudden change in personality, were followed by a major localized seizure.

---

3. A Jacksonian fit is an epileptic seizure (convulsion) which involves a part of the body (not a general one).

My first reaction, once the fit was controlled, was one of guilt at having branded him a troublesome malingerer. Now I had to explain to him and to his wife that the trivial complaint which had so irritated me demanded urgent admission to hospital. There the presence of a rapidly growing glioma, an aggressive brain tumor, was soon confirmed.

To say the least I was somewhat chastened when I reported to my returned partner what had happened. Then George asked a strange thing. "Would you," he asked, "mind taking over the care of John Bradney? Since you started badly perhaps you should have the opportunity to show your true mettle." George paused thoughtfully and added, "I suppose that my real reason for asking is that I have grown so close to that family over the years I am not sure I could cope well with Avis while John is dying of a brain tumor." Despite major misgivings and a firm desire never to meet Mr. Bradney again, I agreed to George's request.

Bradney returned home two months later, after craniotomy[4] and radio-therapy. He had reverted to his normal, pleasant, if somewhat abrasive self who entertained George with their chess games at the farm. He was even apologetic for having been difficult before he went to the hospital, though he had little memory of just how tiresome he had been. However, Avis had told him that the young doctor had been a bit provoked but had done very well in spite of it. This, though somewhat mollifying, brought back my sense of guilt at having so misjudged him. As I left he gave me a brace of pheasants shot by his son that morning. Thus may coals of fire be heaped. As I thanked him he fixed my eye and said, "I rely on you to let me out if it gets too bad. No messing. . . . I want a dose that will finish it."

When I was a medical student we had no teaching about ethics, communication skills, self-awareness, or how to deal with requests like this. Vaguely I nodded and he took this as acquiescence.

By January, despite steroids, his headaches were intense and he was having more frequent fits. I had started morphine and the dose rapidly escalated. One day after a higher than usual dose he died. The family was grateful and relieved; there were more pheasants.

Epilogue

John Bradney taught me much about caring for patients, largely as a result of my own mistakes. Not only did I fail to appreciate the significance of a trivial symptom presented repeatedly by a man who should have been totally absorbed by his harvest, but I allowed my own emotional reaction to block reason. With this realization the new emotion of guilt further complicated my view of the case. This was not helped by the patient's later magnanimity.

Apart from rather nebulous student debates, I had had no teaching and

---

4. A craniotomy is the surgical opening of the skull, in this case to remove the tumor.

thought little about euthanasia. Since then, having worked in the Netherlands and in a hospice, I have thought and taught a great deal about this subject. In consequence I have never acquiesced in euthanasia again. No person wants to die for the sake of being dead, though they may seek relief from the unbearable. The doctor's task is not to kill but to find other ways of relieving the suffering. To do this he must be aware of the totality of that suffering in its psychological, social, and spiritual dimensions as well as the merely physical.

In retrospect, it is doubtful that my patient's death was caused by me. That does not alter the intention behind the act, which was to meet the patient's expressed wish. But the reason behind that wish, with all the complications of a proud man's self-image and the complex relationship with his family and totally dependent wife, remained unexplored. I conceded to his wish; looking back, however, I am sure that I failed him.

Venancio's Legacy

Mario Ahrens

Buenos Aires, Argentina

The old man was sitting on his bed, a bed with a white metal frame and a headboard constructed of tubular cast iron. All of the twenty beds in the large hospital ward were identical and each one had a white cotton bedspread. White had been the original color, but some covers had turned yellow after prolonged use by patients who had lain on these beds. Nevertheless, the place was clean. A strong smell of chlorinated disinfectant permeated the ward. The Hospital de Clinicas was the main teaching hospital for the University of Buenos Aires Medical School and thus it was granted more financial support by the government than other hospitals in the city. The fifty-year-old pavilion had no heating and, in that autumn of 1956, the patients not in bed walked around in woolen overcoats. White sheer screens, mounted on metal frames, provided some privacy to the dying and the seriously ill.

The patient, oblivious to others, was looking through a large paneled window, watching the inner court of the hospital. At age sixty-five, and even after several weeks as an inpatient in that sunless place, Venancio Rocha preserved the dark coloration of his skin, partly inherited from his Spanish, Basque, and Guarano Indian ancestors and partly the result of a long life as a cowhand, a peon, in the Argentine pampa. His brown eyes were like two slits, the effect of squinting in the harsh sun and wind; creases extended from the corner of his eyes to the bushy gray sideburns. Thick gray hair, growing close to his eyebrows, left uncovered a narrow strip of forehead crossed by pale wrinkles; the unexposed furrows contrasted with tanned skin. A drooping mustache almost concealed an easy smile and full lips.

Trying to ignore the back pain that had been nagging him for many weeks, Venancio watched the patio paved with gray flat stones. At places, the pavement was interrupted by circular planters where sycamores grew their grayish trunks. A few yellow and orange leaves still clung to the trees. Like my life, those leaves barely hung on, the old man thought. The scene was very different from his beloved pampa, the plains of Argentina, where he grew up and spent most of his life. Here, one could not see the horizon—buildings crowded the view. There, the vast expanses where the separation of earth and sky was observable for 360 degrees were only rarely interrupted by stands of small native trees or eucalyptus planted close to the houses. But what distressed him most of all was the inability to see the dawns and sunsets—the display of purples, blues, and oranges that was part of the natural harmony of the plains.

Until he was sent to Buenos Aires to be treated, Venancio had never been in the big city. When he arrived he was amazed by the large buildings, the traffic, and the multitudes and annoyed by the cacophony made by cars, trams, and radios. While staying at a boarding house, before being admitted to the hospital, he had committed a mistake that pointed out his ignorance to the "civilized" ways. He had always lived in a house with an earthen floor where spitting the first mouthful of maté,[5] to get rid of the dust in the leaves, was an accepted and necessary habit. When he did the same on the terrazzo floor he was reprimanded by the cook, a short-tempered woman who came from the same province. Venancio wished he were back where he belonged, riding his horse in an early morning, smelling the aroma of thyme in the air, observing the cattle walking slowly in the distance, foraging for fresh grass. Venancio had been a lonely man. His wife Ramona had died many years ago when giving birth to a child. Left a widower without children as a young man, he never remarried. The love for that strong and beautiful woman had been too intense to replace and the pain too severe to forget. Thus, in his usual silent way Venancio Rocha kept working as a peon. The work in the large cattle ranch—*estancia,* as it is called Spanish—had been his life. He had become the foreman of a crew of twenty men that ran the large establishment, more than a hundred thousand acres that belonged to Don Alfonso Etchegaray. His ability as a horseman, his knowledge of the cattle, and his familiarity with the terrain had prompted the respect of his charges and the appreciation of Don Alfonso.

Venancio was a man of short words and long silences. There were a few casual friends, but the only comfort from his loneliness was his friendship with Julio Etchegaray. Julito, as the boy was known, was Don Alfonso's grandson. The child loved the country and admired the old gaucho. During summer vacations, Venancio taught the boy to saddle a horse, to ride, and to understand the many tasks needed to raise cattle. He also showed Julito how to handle the lasso and to hunt ostriches with *boleadoras,* the weapon used by the Pampas Indians.

Sometimes they sat in front of the open fire and, while sipping maté, talked about horses, wild animals and old times when Venancio was a child. He remembered the young boy listening, wide-eyed, to the stories about Venancio's father, how the old man had fought the Pampas Indians in the frontier and how he once escaped to the desert and lived with the same Indians, avoiding political persecution. Venancio missed Julito. The pain in his lower back became more severe as Venancio sat contemplating the yellow leaves piling on the hospital's grounds. He was not a man given to complain. "Pain and suffering is part of life and a man has to learn to accept them," his father had told him after Venancio had fallen from a horse. Very soon they would take him to the building where a strange machine was applied to his

5.   Maté is a tealike drink brewed from leaves and shoots of an evergreen tree; it is popular in South America.

lower back. "Radiation therapy," the doctors had told him, "will kill the cancer growing in your back." Maybe so, he thought, but then what? Six years earlier, Don Alfonso Etchegaray had died. His son Carlos, Julito's father, had little interest in managing the ranch. Wanting the cash, he liquidated the estate, causing Julito great unhappiness. The boy was sixteen at the time and was no longer able to spend his summer vacations in the country. Venancio had lost his spiritual son.

The old foreman never met the new owner. He could not conceive that the land that held so many memories and traditions was owned by a foreign company which only occasionally sent an overseer who lived in the city. The company paid good salaries and took care of its employees, but the special relationship between the "patron" and the peon was gone.

Only a few months before, he noticed that he had to urinate more often, particularly at night. Venancio knew that it was a common complaint among older men and, since he had turned sixty-five, did not pay much attention. A month or so later while riding and rounding up a herd of steers he felt the pain in his lower back that almost immobilized him. And then he could not pass water. Venancio was rushed to the small town where a doctor placed a catheter in his bladder and gave him a thorough examination. He suffered in silence what for a man of his background was the indignity of a rectal exam. "Your prostate is enlarged," the doctor said, "and I don't like that pain in your back." An X-ray showed the tumor growing in his backbone. The manager of the ranch sent him to the city where the medical school was located. Before he left for Buenos Aires, he was told that the large estancia was going to be sold in smaller parcels and Venancio's life, even if he survived the cancer, would never be the same. And then what? He wished he could see Julito again. He had learned that the young man was studying medicine, but he doubted he would find the medical student in this maze of corridors and buildings.

"Venancio Rocha!" The voice of the male medical assistant brought him back from his ruminations, "It's time to go for therapy."

Julio Etchegaray was walking through the long corridor that led into the urology ward. The tousle-haired young man was lean and of medium height. He had an engaging smile that contrasted with the sadness of his eyes; the outer corners pointed slightly down. While walking toward the ward, where he was assigned to take a history and physical exam, he thought about his studies and the task ahead of him. After two years in medical school he was not sure he had chosen the right path. He loved life in the open, the unbounded freedom of the pampa, the sunsets, the lagoons with flamingos, and he enjoyed working with the herd of cattle, the way Venancio had taught him. The feeling of wind on his face as he rode his horse at full gallop, and the clear and crispy nights, when the dark sky was speckled with brilliant dots, were experiences he could not forget.

Being a cattle rancher would have been his first choice, but then his grandfather had died and his father sold the land. Confronted by the need to choose a profession and by the family who demanded a university title, he had chosen to study medicine. An avid reader, Julito had read *The Citadel* by A. J. Cronin as well as Frank Slaughter's *Men in White,* and the selfless, dedicated characters in these novels had impressed his young soul. In his romantic notions he wanted to be like them, healing and alleviating suffering, but the first two years in medical school were disappointing. It seemed the learning of biological sciences and the applied methods to fight diseases—the long hours spent in the anatomy lab, the intricacies of physiology and bacteriology, the memorization of symptoms and syndromes—took precedence over the spiritual side of medicine. But by simple inertia and habit of studying, Julio kept moving forward, if only with mediocre grades and lukewarm enthusiasm. As he approached the waiting room in front of the ward, Julio saw an old man sitting on a wooden bench. There was something familiar about his posture. The man was sitting straight as if riding a horse and looking through a window; his squinting eyes were pointed far beyond the narrow hospital court. Julio recognized the graying hair and the drooping mustache. "Venancio!" he shouted, elated by the encounter, and gave the old man a hug. "Julito, I hoped I would find you here."

"Why are you in this hospital, so far away from home?"

The old man told the medical student about his symptoms and what he had heard from the doctors, even when he did not always understood their explanations.

"Let's go out to the court where we have privacy," Julio said, helping the old gaucho to walk. Venancio concealed his pain but could not stretch his right leg. Assisted by Julio, he walked with a limp to a park bench where they both sat in the mild autumn afternoon among the pigeons near the statue of an old professor, the founder of the hospital.

"Remember when you were chased by a cow during that round-up?" Venancio asked with a big smile.

"Yes, I remember. I was twelve years old and trying to brand the calf when the angry mother charged me."

"You ran faster than an ostrich." Venancio was now laughing, maybe for the first time in many weeks. So they went on remembering the old times when the foreman helped the child to grow up and taught him to be a cowhand. After that reunion, Julio visited the patient every day. He reviewed the chart and understood the gravity of the prognosis, and his hopes—born out of lack of experience—were soon destroyed by the chief resident, who told him that his old friend would die in a few weeks. He could see it himself.

Every day Venancio looked thinner and his brown skin was turning olive. Julio brought food from home and tried to feed him, but most important, they kept reminiscing. In all that time Venancio never complained or showed signs of pain. It was a moving experience for Julio, who tried hard to cheer up his old friend and mentor.

Two weeks later, while Julio was visiting—as he always did before morning lectures—two senior medical students came by the bedside.

"We are going to examine the patient," one said with authoritative voice.

"What for?" Julio asked.

"We need to check his prostate to see how large it has become."

Julio moved away from the bed and, taking both students by their arms forced them a few yards away from where Venancio was resting.

"Look," he said in a soft voice, "the man is dying. Leave him alone."

"Either you move away or I will report you to the chief resident," the older student retorted.

Julio's eyes narrowed and his face turned pale. His full lips became tight lines and his shoulders were drawn back. "Get out of here or fight me." His voice was sibilant and his fists were tight.

The senior students, not wanting confrontation with this angry man, left the room.

Venancio was comatose, but Julio noticed a hint of a smile under the drooping mustache.

As he was dying, the old gaucho saw himself on his gray mare driving hundreds of heads; he could feel the gritty dirt in his teeth and hear the bawling of the cows and the whistling of the cowhands; over there, pushing the herd, he saw a tousle-haired boy riding a bay gelding. Then, slowly, the lights went out and the Impenetrable Silence set in. Julio placed his stethoscope on his old friend's chest and confirmed that there were no sounds. He pushed the eyelids shut and then walked to the nurses' desk. Pronouncing Venancio Rocha dead, Julio signed the chart. With his fist—almost in anger—he wiped a tear from his cheek.

His white gown flowing in a wintry breeze, his stethoscope still hanging from his neck, Julio walked the short distance that separated the hospital from the university, where he had to attend a lecture. He was thinking of his dead friend and, in his sadness, he found consolation. He had comforted the old man in his last days. During that short walk he began to realize that he had performed part of the physician's mission. He had loved the old man, and that love was being transferred to the many patients he would encounter in his professional life. There would be many Venancios in need of care and warmth; some he would be able to heal, many he would console and palliate. Thus his vision of what medicine should be was met for the first time.

Gradually he was falling in love for the second time. The first love had been with the open plains and the country life; the second was with a more demanding and exacting mistress. Medicine was going to be his lover for the rest of his life. The two passions in Julio's life were Venancio's legacy.

Epilogue

Julio Etchegaray is a pseudonym I have chosen. Like Julio, I was a reluctant medical student. I had spent many summers on my grandfather's ranch and wanted to be a cattleman, but societal and family demands prompted my attending medical school. The sad event described in the story, the death of an old cowhand named Venancio who worked for my family, occurred while I was a medical student. The experience slowly changed my mind about my vocation.

The Promise: A Love Story

Perle Feldman

Montreal, Quebec

I first met the Jacksons ten years ago. I had taken over a practice from a physician who had made a point of transferring these special people to me. At that time Mr. Jackson's health was of great concern. He was suffering from scleroderma, a horrible autoimmune disease where the body treats its own tissue as foreign, and attacks it. The normal body tissue is slowly replaced by scar tissue, and the patient is progressively less able to move. Mr. Jackson had the most serious form of scleroderma, where the lungs are the primary target. His lungs were being changed into fibrous sacs by the attack of his own misguided immune system, and he was slowly strangling to death.

A few months after I had met them, when Mr. Jackson had just come out of the hospital, I went to have a home visit with him. They lived in a veterans' apartment building not far from my office. Mr. Jackson sat in his big armchair, tied by his oxygen tank and nasal prongs. His skin was abnormally smooth. He looked somewhat like a statue of Buddha, but with the hawklike profile of a Canadian aboriginal. His breath was harsh and his lips were drawn and blue. I checked his lungs. The sound of his breathing reminded me of someone popping the bubbles in bubble wrap. The sound was unbelievable. I called his respiratory specialist. "What should I do for him?" I asked. "I don't know," said his specialist. " He should be dead in a month or two. There's not much anyone can do at this point." Consequently, I attended to the dying of Mr. Jackson. I saw Mrs. Jackson quite frequently. She was very stressed and not sleeping much; listening to her husband gasp and choke beside her was not restful. Her blood pressure was not in great control, something I attributed to stress. Her only respite was the hour or two she spent downstairs in the recreation hall of the building, playing cards and smoking cigarette after cigarette.

Over the next few months I learned a lot about the history of the Jackson family. They had met in Holland. Young Angus Jackson was a soldier in the Canadian army during the liberation of Holland. He had met his bride when she defied her parents and went to a dance at the base. They courted during that heady postwar time. He was a Native Canadian from Saskatchewan—"a real red Indian," Alice called him. Alice was a well brought up Dutch girl with a crown of braids and a bicycle. Somehow they fell in love and decided to marry, even though they shared less than fifty words in a common language. Against her parents' wishes she followed him to Canada, where they married and went off to a remote section of rural Saskatchewan.

The Jacksons had seven children. The first was born on the remote farm where they were living and working. It was the middle of winter. When Alice's labor began Angus left to get the wife of the farmer and got caught in a snowstorm. Alice labored for hours alone and in pain. She told me she was so innocent and ignorant she had no idea where the baby would come out. When her waters broke she thought she had wet herself. When the baby started to emerge she was hanging onto the head of the iron bedstead, screaming. Her first reaction was total surprise to see the dark haired head emerge from between her legs. By the time Angus returned with help she had already managed to clean the baby up and cut the cord herself. "Look, you have a son," she said as he walked in the door.

They lived through good times and bad, with seven children to bring them joy and trouble. Sometimes they had no money, sometimes Angus drank too much, but somehow the incandescent flame of love which had started in Holland became the warmth of a family. Through it all they survived together.

They would not be together much longer. Angus was fading, although he held tenaciously to life. It took more and more effort to drag air in and out of his stiff lungs. After four months he was still alive. I talked to him about his arrangements; he had no will and had a superstition about making one. "Just write me a letter" I begged him. "Just write to me and say that you want to leave everything to your wife." But I don't think he ever did.

Alice came to my office every two weeks or so. I would play with her blood pressure medication, listen to her troubles, and let her cry. One day she came in with a numb, cold, left hand. When I examined her she had no radial pulse in her forearm because her subclavian artery, the blood vessel under her collarbone, was blocked. I sent her up to the hospital for some tests. They wanted to keep her but she insisted on going home because she couldn't leave Angus. Eventually she recovered, leaving just a slight weakness in that hand and a diminished pulse in that arm.

As Angus continued to fade, Alice's exhaustion became obvious. She was looking really thin. I suggested putting him into the hospital for a few weeks, just so that she could get some rest. Angus did not want to go back into the hospital. "If they ever get me back in there," he said, "I'll never walk out again. I want to die here in my own home, in my own chair." "We've been together for forty years," Alice said, "I'll not leave him now." I finally convinced her to call her children and ask for help. Until now she had refused to even do this. The daughters and sons living in Montreal began to spend time at the apartment, allowing Alice a little rest.

One morning, just as I came in to work, I got the call. It was Mrs. Jackson: "Can you come right away, he looks awful bad." I grabbed my home visit bag and ran over. When I got there her neighbors were waiting for me in the lobby. They escorted me upstairs in an oddly formal way. As I got out of the elevator they hung back. I knocked on the door. Mrs. Jackson opened it, her face convulsed with sorrow. "He's gone Perle, Gus is gone."

I entered the neat apartment filled with the memorabilia of forty years of married life. Angus was sitting in his chair and was indeed dead. I made the formal examination of his heart and breathing. I closed his mouth and eyes and removed his oxygen. I turned to Mrs. Jackson and shook my head. "He's gone Alice." She cried harshly and I held onto her. The neighbors slowly began to come into the apartment. Her son and daughter burst through the door and stopped suddenly, as they realized they were too late. Someone made tea. A friend phoned The Last Post, an organization which cares for the burial of veterans. I filled out a death certificate. Angus had gotten his wish; he had died in his own chair and Alice had fulfilled her promise to him. She completed their life together with love, honor, and fidelity.

Jaw Pain and Panic: What to Do When Patients Consulting You Die in the Seat Belt

Ivar Ostergaard
Galten, Denmark

About ten years ago, the phone rang when I was just beginning an on-call duty. A stressed husband asked if I would take a look at his wife, who was having severe pain in her jaw. She was moaning loudly in the background, racked with pain. She was in her late sixties, previously in good health "but she is in such pain—please take a look and help her!" She had just been discharged from the hospital after five days, having had attacks of the pain for some weeks. Lots of tests had been done, but they had all turned out normal. No diagnosis had been made, and no clear explanation provided, except that the attacks of pain might be due to some kind of neuritis. We agreed that they would come and meet me at the clinic right away

When she arrived, she was still in pain and looked pale, with cool, sweaty skin, fearful, and in distress. After apologizing for disturbing me, she pleaded, "Please help me to get rid of the pain." A detailed history revealed that the attacks of pain started abruptly, without any definable provoking factors. The pain was located in her jaw without radiation to her chest, although she had some sensations down her neck. The pain was "oppressive" and "squeezing." Although she was not nauseated, she complained of "sweating all over" and of having a strange feeling in her cheeks. She was also a little short of breath. She had never had any problems with her heart or any other health problems.

Her appearance and the oppressive nature of her pain made me think about angina pectoris.[6] We did an electrocardiogram, which showed signs of cardiac ischemia, supporting my suspicion. Receiving a diagnosis satisfied her and she was even more content when she was immediately relieved by her first dose of nitroglycerine. "How wonderful you could figure out what it is! Now that I know what it's all about, I am sure I can manage the pain."

She jumped off the couch and was ready to leave, looking well with no trouble moving around. A prescription was written for nitroglycerine tablets and after a few minutes, off the couple went to the pharmacy. I felt good, having made the proper diagnosis and having relieved my patient of her pain.

Less than ten minutes later her husband came in the back door, a little pale but calm, and said: "I think my wife is dead!" I went outside and discovered her sitting in the front seat of the car, dead indeed, well beyond reach of CPR (cardiopulmonary resuscitation). He received this news in a state of calm

---

6. Angina pectoris is a severe constricting pain in the chest caused by lack of blood flow to the heart muscle.

shock. The story was that they had driven the short distance to the pharmacy, chatting about how well things would be from now on, now that they knew what the problem was. The husband went in to buy the medication; he was gone for no more than five minutes when he returned to the car to find his wife showing no sign of life. He turned the car around and raced to the clinic, driving to the back entrance; he wanted "to be discrete, if she was really dead."

After receiving my confirmation that his wife was dead, he asked a practical question: "What to do next?" My thoughts were racing: Had I just committed malpractice? Had I just made a major mistake? I felt somewhat assured that she had gotten well after one dose of nitroglycerine, that the complaints had been there for some time, and that she had just been discharged from the hospital. But what to do with the corpse? If we lifted her out of the car and into the clinic, I would be tied up for hours and could not attend other patients. Calling the emergency unit would be very inappropriate . . . but would it be appropriate to drive her back home, sitting in the front seat? There we could lift her out of the car and lay her in her own bed. Without knowing how exactly we arrived at this point, we agreed to take her home, keeping her in the front seat with the seat belt secured. Did the event and circumstances dictate what could and should be done? I don't know. We called for a son living nearby to help us. He agreed without hesitation and strangely enough, like his father, he acted as if the young doctor on call had made a good decision. When we arrived at the house a neighbor helped to carry her into the bedroom. Family members gathered and I left with mixed feelings I still vividly remember today. What had I experienced? Were the husband and the son in shock and therefore unable to judge my actions, or did they manifest an acceptance of death as a natural part of life to be "handled practically." Were my decisions and deeds after the death guided by clever judgment, insensitivity, panic, or were they just reflex actions in a very unusual situation?

I will never know. . . .

However, should there be a next time I will call a deputy, arrange for alternative transportation, and stay with the family longer.

The surviving family members are still patients of mine!

Mr. Jones Needs to Be DNR'ed

Kurt C. Stange
Cleveland, Ohio

At "morning report" the resident physician on call overnight reports on patients who were admitted to the hospital or who suffered a change in status. Dr. Oliver matter-of-factly recounted the details of Mr. Jones's admission.

"Mr. Jones is a seventy-eight-year-old African American male transferred to the hospital last night because of a pneumonia that had been unresponsive to treatment with oral antibiotics at the nursing home. His past medical history is significant for severe dementia and hypertension. . . ."

The rest of the presentation depicted the details of a man who was unable to care for himself or to interact with the rest of the world in a meaningful way. He was now in the midst of a new illness that had the potential to take his life. Mr. Jones was just the sort of man that the great physician Sir William Osler was referring to when he called pneumonia, with its fatal potential, "the old man's friend."

Dr. Oliver continued his presentation: "Mr. Jones had been a 'DNR' at the nursing home until last week, when his wife changed her mind and made him 'full code.' I called her last night, and she wouldn't change her mind, insisting that we make all efforts to resuscitate her husband if his heart or breathing stopped. I told her about the futility of resuscitation, but she just wouldn't listen to reason."

Muffled groans and murmurs of sympathy were emitted from the assembled physicians and students. "DNR" means "do not resuscitate." Getting patient's or family members' permission for DNR orders is a high priority for any physician who has gone through the painful exercise of performing cardiopulmonary resuscitation, mechanical ventilation, electrical cardioversion, and the other routines of attempting to revive a person whose condition makes these efforts futile. A consensus emerged that the resident taking over the patient's care and I, as the attending physician, should prevail upon the patient's wife to listen to reason and consent to the DNR status. The medical team was greatly satisfied to learn that the night resident had arranged a meeting for that afternoon, in which Mr. Jones's wife would come into the hospital to discuss the situation with us.

Soon the call arrived from the nurse that Mrs. Jones was here to visit her husband. As the day resident, Dr. Nagel, and I walked up the hospital floor, we concurred that most people are reasonable. Mrs. Jones's apparently unreasonable behavior might have a reasonable basis, if we could find a way to understand things from her perspective. We decided to try to understand, instead of, or at least prior to, trying to persuade.

When we entered the room, Mr. Jones appeared gravely ill. Still breathing heavily, he brushed back our attempts to talk to him or to listen to his lungs. He had refused all attempts by the nurses to feed him, and he was incontinent of both bladder and bowels. Surely, if his infected lungs or frail heart should fail, resuscitation would have a less than 1 percent chance of succeeding. In any case, was this a life worth saving?

Mrs. Jones entered the room. Without pausing for introductions, she rushed over and kissed her husband. Tenderly, he kissed her back. A warm embrace ensued, followed by a repartee of sweet nothings that would have been embarrassing in a young couple but were touching in their ability to communicate deep feelings of affection between a husband who couldn't speak coherent sentences and his loving wife. A single tear of happiness rolled down Mr. Jones's cheek. Many more tears welled up in the eyes of the two doctors who were privileged observers of the interaction.

Mrs. Jones chided: "I hear you haven't been eating for these nice people. What are you trying to do, starve yourself to death? Come on, I need you around to keep me company."

Slowly but steadily, Mr. Jones gummed and swallowed each spoonful proffered by Mrs. Jones. During the meal, we asked Mrs. Jones about her life with Mr. Jones. After fifty years filled with many struggles, and an equal portion of joys and tragedies, Mr. Jones had suffered a series of strokes that left him mentally diminished. Nursing home placement was the only option to care for his needs, but Mrs. Jones visited him each day. He had lived a full life, and consistent with her understanding of what his wishes would be, she had readily agreed to DNR orders at the nursing home. However, when he became ill, Mrs. Jones found that do not resuscitate orders are often equivalent to the instruction "do not care." Help with eating, dressing, and toileting were minimally offered, and Mrs. Jones's visits became painful exercises in watching unrequited suffering. Transferring care to a new group of strangers, Mrs. Jones didn't want another "do not care" order.

"Would you want your husband to receive electric shocks to the chest if his heart should stop beating?"

"Of course not."

"How about putting him on a breathing machine if he should stop breathing on his own?"

"Not unless we're sure he could stop the machine soon and still live. I just want any infection to be treated, and help with getting him to eat and use the toilet."

"We can do that."

A few moments of seeking to understand has had a profound effect. Almost incidentally, the patient's wife had agreed to the DNR status. More profoundly for Dr. Nagel and me, the privilege of watching Mr. and Mrs. Jones's tender interactions had reminded us of the value of life, even life in a muted and diminished appearance. It had also taught us a lesson in humility and the power of love, loyalty, and devotion.

References

Balint, M. 1952. *The Doctor, His Patient and the Illness.* New York: International Universities Press.

Cassell, E. J. 1985. *Talking with Patients.* Cambridge, Mass.: MIT Press.

Cole-Kelly, K. 1994. Illness stories and patient care in the family practice context. *Family Medicine.* 2(1):45–48.

Field, M. and Cassel, K. (eds.). 1997. *Approaching Death: Improving Care at the End of Life.* Washington, D.C.: National Academy Press.

McDaniel, S., J. Hepworth, and W. Doherty. 1992. *Medical Family Therapy.* New York: Basic Books.

McDaniel, S., T. Campbell, and D. Seaburn. 1993. *Family Oriented Primary Care.* New York: Springer-Verlag.

Imber-Black, E., J. Roberts, and R. Whiting. *Rituals in Family Therapy.* New York: Norton.

Secrets

Reflections

Aya Biderman, Jeffrey M. Borkan, and Shmuel Reis

Secrets—the common theme of the five stories in this chapter—manifest themselves in very different kinds of concealed or shrouded truth, yet in each story the secret has an important role and its revelation represents a turning point in the physician's contact with the patient or with the patient's family. One might first associate the notion of "secrets in medicine" with doctors' difficulty or hesitancy to share "bad news" or "exclusive information" with patients or others. A more accurate picture, however, is that participation in keeping, maintaining, and revealing secrets is bipartisan, involving both patients and physicians.

The rich patchwork of encounters in this chapter weaves together themes of distance and closeness, boundaries and dependence. Guilt, shame, and responsibility are exemplified through narratives of marital conflict and abuse, homosexuality, and suicide. The stories bring to mind the emotions and fears felt by physicians, students, patients, and their respective significant others regarding lies, disclosure, truth, and timing. Many practitioners have heard their patients report vague unexplained symptoms and interpreted these as somatic "admission tickets" meant to bring the encounter to what "really matters." Many others, both patient and provider, have told, been told, or suspected harmful secrets, challenging secrets, "secrets of the couch and the grave" (Pellegrino 1996).

Every patient has his or her own story of illness, his or her particular ways of coming to terms with loss, sorrow, joy, and his or her own secrets. Burnum (1991) describes the secrets revealed to him over a fourteen-year period of medical practice and divides them into categories: injurious personal habits, mental or physical incapacity, family discord, and hidden physical symptoms. A family therapy approach has been adopted by Imber-Black (1993), who categorizes secrets into three groups: positive, toxic, and dangerous. Positive secrets are those that are normative, such as not telling relatives about a new pregnancy until after the first trimester. Toxic secrets are those that make the family members distrust each other, such as concealing a difficult diagnosis from the patient. Dangerous secrets are those that require the health professional to act immediately to prevent further risk for the patient or family members involved, for instance, the revelation of ongoing physical or sexual abuse.

When we, as health care providers, get a very important piece of information that was kept from us for a long time, we often ask ourselves, "Why didn't he tell me before?" Among the multiple reasons and motivations for patients to hold onto secrets are the following:

- The patient thinks that the information is not relevant to the problem.
- The physician does not "make it possible" for the patient to feel secure enough to reveal the secret.
- The secret provides the patient with a sense of power and control; holding onto the secret leaves the patient in charge.
- The secret is associated with feelings of guilt or shame and the patient may be concerned that its knowledge will cause the physician to lower his or her opinion of the patient.
- The secret concerns an issue with criminal or legal ramifications.
- The secret involves conflicts of interest.

When looking at this list, it is clear that not only patients' secrets are at stake— each item can apply to physicians' secrets as well. Health care providers' secrets, particularly those of nondisclosure, are common. Only a generation ago, American physicians rarely told their patients that they had cancer, while Italian, Japanese, and many other nations' doctors still continue to mask or withhold the diagnosis (GIVIO 1986; Munakata 1986; Good 1990). Such nondisclosure is often justified in terms of maintaining "hope" (Good 1990), assisting in the care of the patient, or protecting the patient.

Secrets hold power. Secrets held by patients or providers may be a means by which they maintain control, whether in the context of the individual, the family, the society, or the provider–patient relationship. (For example, in Dr. Summer's story, does the secret "protect" just the doctor's wife, or does it also protect the doctor's emotional state and sense of control?) A common secret creates a sense of togetherness by dividing *us* from *them*. Conversely, "letting go" of secrets is sometimes painful and frightening. It might mean giving up strength and charge. It might also mean letting somebody into the intimacy of the family or the intricacies of the medical profession, breaking the walls between "us" and "them."

Secrets also satisfy the need for confiding. There are good reasons to create an environment and a therapeutic relationship in which patients can reveal their secrets. The psychotherapist Susan Baur (1995) uses the term *confiding* for the special kind of storytelling about misfortunes that happen to people: death of loved ones, diseases, sexual abuse, and so on. By confiding in another person, the individual who experiences the loss not only receives more support, but also suffers fewer health problems and reacts better to stress than those who do not confide (Baur 1995). Toombs (1992) has described the need for the differing worlds of the patient and the physician to engage in the doctor–patient encounter in order for a healing relationship to be possible. Secrets, concealment, and shrouded mysteries might well be considered impediments to healing. In psychoanalysis, the revelation of secrets is at the core of the psychotherapeutic method, and is even "regarded as the seed from which early psychoanalytic theory grew" (Mears 1976). There is also an important role for secrets in the provider–patient relationship in general and family practice. For some people, the primary care physician is the only confidant for certain issues. Balint (1973) described "flashes" which occurred in such settings. These flashes are moments of revelation—sometimes of a secret, always of an understanding. Balint believed that such revelations should be cherished, acknowledged silently by patient and physician as the crucible of healing.

Some of the storytellers in this chapter share with us such moments. The flashes may have occurred during the first encounter as in Dr. Stange's case, or after twelve years when "it's safe enough to believe that you will stick around" for Dr. Herbert. They are often preceded by futile biomedical searches, as in Dr. Rosser's story where the clues hid thirty-five years of suffering. This last case also demonstrates the importance of the family physician as the confidant, to whom telling the secret may change the whole view.

The revelation of secrets may create new issues for provider and patient. For example, conflicts of interest may occur when the patient asks the provider not to disclose some newly provided information to the family or, in cases where there is a legal requirement, to governmental agencies. How does a doctor react when a patient does not want to tell his or her spouse a new diagnosis of HIV? How does a doctor manage a situation where a spouse does not want the abuse against her to be reported to the police or social services? Particularly in family medicine, the issue becomes, "Who is the patient?" "To whom to be true, the patient, the family, or the greater community or society?"

Secrets are just one kind of barrier in communication between doctors and patients. As Quill (1989) has written, these barriers exist and we must learn to deal with them. The first step is to realize that there is a barrier; then the doctor and the patient, working together, can try to overcome it. In tandem with the current "patient-centered clinical method" (Stewart et al. 1995), as providers we may need to accept that the patient in front of us controls the information, he is the one who will decide what to say and what to keep away from his doctor. As providers we must wait patiently, with an open eye and a listening heart, for the time to arrive. As secret keepers, we must consider when that role is appropriate, and when it merely protects us or our professional hegemony and power.

The Hidden Patient: An Incident
That Changed My Professional Life

Jack H. Medalie
Ni Ya, Israel

"Doctor, nurse Sarah asks that you come quickly. Something bad happened at the Ackermans' home." That was the entreaty by the man standing at our door at two on a winter's night. Telling him that I would come immediately, I dressed warmly, took my doctor's bag, and rushed to my jeep.

On the way to the nearby farming settlement in rural Israel (about twelve kilometers over a rough, muddy road) I had time to reflect about the Ackermans. Almost two months earlier, a middle-aged couple had moved from their cooperative settlement (kibbutz) to Ni Ya, one of the five agricultural settlements that I served as a physician. The husband had suffered a myocardial infarction and had been hospitalized for three weeks. On discharge, he and his wife had come straight to their new apartment on the Ni Ya settlement, which I visited every week for two four- to five-hour sessions (in addition to being on twenty-four-hour call for emergencies). The settlement had a resident nurse (Sarah), who was experienced and efficient. I knew that if she called me in the middle of the night, it must be an emergency, so I responded without asking the messenger for any details. I had visited Mr. Ackerman in his apartment almost every time I worked at Ni Ya—a total of about ten home visits to his place before that emergency call. Each time, I found no evidence of any complications. However, he continued to complain of weakness and lightheadedness. Despite the efforts of his wife, the nurse, and me, he spent most of the day in bed or sitting in a chair. At each visit, his wife was present and asked detailed questions about diet, sleep, bowel habits, and the like, often writing down my answers. She struck me as a somewhat obsessive person who was dedicated to the well-being of her husband, despite his somewhat irritating dependence on others.

During the drive, I kept visualizing different scenarios. Mr. Ackerman had a recurrent infarct,[1] or perhaps I had missed a cardiac aneurysm[2] that had burst. Had he perhaps developed a deep vein thrombosis[3] in his legs from inactivity and shot a pulmonary embolus?[4] All my scenarios ended in Mr. A

1. A recurrent infarct is a repeat heart attack with damage to the heart muscle.
2. A cardiac aneurysm is a thinning or bulging of a weakened wall of a cardiac ventricle (a chamber of the heart), usually caused by a heart attack.
3. A deep vein thrombosis is a blood clot in a large vein of the leg.
4. A pulmonary embolus is a blood clot that wedges in an artery of the lungs, usually a fragment from clots in the leg or pelvis.

being in extremis, if not dead. My own anxiety was high by the time I reached their apartment.

As I entered, the first person I noticed was Mr. Ackerman—to my amazement, he was standing up. He came quickly over to me and whispered, "I'm all right, it's my wife!" Nurse Sarah then quickly took me by the arm and led me into the next room where Mrs. Ackerman was stretched out on the bed. I was dimly aware of Sarah talking to me as I bent over and concentrated on the battered, blood-spattered person on the bed. It took only a few moments to realize that she was dead. Then Sarah's message came into focus— Mrs. Ackerman had committed suicide by throwing herself off a nearby cliff!

Although many years have passed since the incident, I still get a strange feeling when thinking about it. I had been to the Ackermans' home numerous times, always concentrating on the biomedical aspects of the man who had a myocardial infarction, never paying attention to or noticing the person who was really in need of help!

Following the autopsy and funeral (which the husband attended) there was a mourning period of a week and then the husband (the same man who until then had only reluctantly left his bed) returned to his usual occupation of driving a tractor or plow on the farm for a full working day!

All this wreaked havoc with my self-confidence. First I had missed noticing the really sick person. Second, the original patient, whom I had been unable to get to move from his bed, now, following his wife's death, had returned spontaneously to a full working day. My good biomedical education had not helped me. I had completely missed the dysfunctional family relationship!

The next event in this saga occurred about two weeks later. It was the custom then that on every other Friday morning many community physicians would accompany the chairman of the Department of Internal Medicine on ward rounds at the nearby university hospital. Following the round, we adjourned to a small conference room where one or two community physicians would present interesting "cases" for discussion. At the meeting following the suicide incident, I told the story of the "A" couple. There was a short hushed silence, then the professor, presumably trying to be kind to me, said, "Dr. Medalie, don't be so upset. After all, the woman was not your patient!"

Epilogue

The professor's support did not make me feel much better and the incident occupied my thinking for a long time. After recovering from the shock, I started asking myself what lessons could be learned from this experience. What changes could I introduce to my practice so that this type of thing would not recur?

Eventually I became a dedicated proponent of what George Engel (1977) called the biopsychosocial model of disease and medical practice, fully believing that the understanding and treatment of individual patients demand the widening of the biomedical areas to include emotional and social aspects. After much thought, the "hidden patient" concept crystallized: in any family in which there is an individual with an acute and life-threatening or chronic and long-term illness or disease, the caregiver (usually the spouse, the oldest daughter, or sometimes the whole family unit) is under considerable stress. Unless this caregiver receives sufficient support from the family and/or others, coping mechanisms will fail, and the caregiver will develop overt or covert signs of illness—from duodenal ulcers, hypertension, and migraine to heart attacks, strokes, and even death (Medalie 1975, 1994). The prevention of these conditions and the promotion of the health of the caregiver are receiving increased attention of many health and allied disciplines (Kahana, Biegel, and Wykle 1994). The unfortunate incident in this story was what some call their "ah-ha" experience. It certainly changed my way of thinking and practicing medicine for all time.

A Hidden Fear

Kurt C. Stange
Cleveland, Ohio

It was 4:55 P.M. on Friday afternoon. I grabbed the chart of the last patient to be seen and glanced at the chief complaint written by the medical assistant: "New patient. Follow-up of staple in thumb, seen last week in the emergency room."

"Great," I said to the fourth-year medical student who was accompanying me that day. "This should be quick, and we'll get out of here on time for once. How about if we see this patient together? You take the history, and I'll just watch."

"OK," said the student, apparently glad for this time-saving opportunity to have his history-taking skills observed. We entered the room, to be greeted by a forty-year-old, apparently anxious, man.

"Good afternoon, Mr. Ceznic. I'm a student doctor working with Dr. Stange."

The patient looked even more anxious.

"Tell us what brings you here today."

"I accidentally got a staple in my thumb last week. I took it out myself, but went to the emergency room to get it checked. They told me to follow up here with you."

"Is it bothering you at all?"

"No."

"Is there anything else you'd like us to check on while you're here today?"

I was pleased that the student sensed that there might be some other reason for the visit besides this trivial complaint that seemed to be of little concern to the patient.

Mr. Ceznic squirmed in his chair. He looked back and forth between the student and me, as if trying to decide if it was safe to proceed. Finally, quietly, he said, "Yes. I think I may have a urine infection."

"What makes you think that?"

"Sometimes, it hurts a little when I urinate and I have to go more often."

"How long has this been going on?"

"Two weeks."

Having come to the end of his standard questions for urinary tract infections without receiving any suggestive information, the student looked back at me, as if asking for help. I continued eliciting the medical history, taking the questioning in a different direction that might help to explain Mr. Ceznic's roundabout way of bringing up this issue.

"Mr. Ceznic, are you sexually active?"

"Yes."

"With one, or more than one partner?"

He stared at his shoes as he responded, "I guess you could say more than one."

"Men, women, or both?"

A wave of redness rushed up from his neck to the top of his head, and the veins on his forehead bulged, as Mr. Ceznic blurted out: "Both!"

As we kept on talking, the whole story came out. Mr. Ceznic had been faithfully married for twenty years. He had had homosexual feelings since adolescence, even telling his wife about them before they were married. He had never acted on those feelings—that is, until two weeks ago. He had been on a business trip out of town on his fortieth birthday. After a couple of celebratory drinks at the bar at his hotel, he began conversing with another man. He hadn't asked his name, but they ended up back in his hotel room, engaging in oral sex. Mr. Ceznic said that he regretted this lapse in his customary lifestyle, and he had no desire to leave his marriage or act out his occasional homosexual feelings. However, he had hardly slept since the incident. He said he was scared to death that he had gotten AIDS and was risking infecting his wife and children. He had avoided having sex with his wife since the episode but was running out of excuses, and he felt that he had to tell her what had happened.

As our conversation progressed, I happened to look over the medical student, whose presence both Mr. Ceznic and I had temporarily forgotten. The student was sitting upright, stiff as a board, his knuckles white as the paper on the exam table. He later told me that he wished he could have found a hole to crawl into, but there was nowhere to hide.

I reassured Mr. Ceznic about the relatively low risk of transmitting HIV during a single episode of oral sex, even with a high-risk partner. We discussed the negligible risk of transmission to his children and options for minimizing the risk of transmission to his wife until his own HIV status was clarified. He agreed to serial HIV testing. Armed with this information, he volunteered that he would tell his wife. I offered to be there when he told her and suggested that we schedule a follow-up visit to discuss both of their concerns. I also offered to arrange a session with a professional counselor, where we could discuss his sexual orientation, guilt, and other feelings.

Mr. Ceznic decided to get anonymous HIV testing at the local free clinic. He tested negative that evening and six weeks later. I saw him for two follow-up visits, both of them by himself. He said that he had told his wife the evening of the first visit to me, and that she was both understanding and forgiving. To my disappointment, Mr. Ceznic never brought his wife in to see me, and after his six-week follow-up visit, I never saw him again either. I was disappointed because I thought that I could be most helpful by getting to know both of them. Clearly, they were both affected by this incident and its underlying causes. Moreover, I wanted to meet this woman, who was apparently saintlike in her forgiveness and understanding, to see if she was real.

Tincture of Time

Carol P. Herbert

Vancouver, British Columbia

I met C. G. during my first year in practice in a health center located in an urban area of Canada, populated by the working poor and families on social welfare. She was a young single mother, depressed and unemployed, with a one-year old boy. She had grown up in foster care with a white family, with limited contact with her First Nations (Native Indian) parents, who lived on the reservation. The father of C. G.'s child was a married Jamaican man who had beaten her on more than one occasion.

When C. G. attempted suicide, I supported her through recovery. When necessary, I went to court to help her regain custody of her child from the child protection agency. My professional boundaries were definitely more permeable than usual with this woman, whose need for unconditional love and support was stronger than her need for biomedical treatment. I gave her my home number and talked her down from crises. I felt that if we could build a relationship of trust and respect, she might be able to move through this period of her life and find some peace. I encouraged her to write poetry and to share her imagery of "the land of darkness" in which she found herself so often. I tried to understand the context of the pain that drove her into such deep depression. Sometimes, I confess, I wanted to distance myself because I did not know what to say or do to "make it better." I was afraid she would kill herself and that I would feel it was my fault, because I had not treated her vigorously enough for her psychiatric symptoms. Intuitively, I felt that admission to the psychiatry ward would be more for my sake than for hers; I would be less afraid, but she would be confirmed in the belief that she was "sick," "weak," and "dependent."

During this time I felt certain that C. G. had been abused as a child, but she denied this during my screening questions. It was hard to let go of the need to confirm my suspicions and the desire to be a "good diagnostician," who could "cure" her. But I did back off my questioning.

Twelve years into our patient–physician relationship, during a routine visit, C. G. disclosed the sexual and psychological abuse which she suffered at the hands of her foster father.

C. G. knew that I had special interest and training in child sexual abuse and family violence, yet she waited twelve years to share her secret. When I asked why she had decided to disclose this information during this visit, she replied, "When I first met you, I didn't know if I could trust you. Then after awhile, I got to depend on you and on your liking me. I was afraid that you would reject me if you knew who I really was. It's taken till now to get to the point where I feel safe enough with you to believe that you will stick around."

Epilogue

Was I right in not forcing the issue earlier in our relationship? Did my attempts to screen for a history of family violence help to set the stage for her disclosure when she felt ready? Could I have done something else to make her feel safe enough to disclose the issues years before? Is there a "right time" for disclosure? The answers are not simple. I believe that if I had forced disclosure, I would have broken trust and damaged that fragile, precious sense of self-worth and internal ability to control her life that she was beginning to experience. It was only within a longstanding relationship with me as caregiver, supporter, advocate, coach, and friend that she was able to heal enough to feel that she could let her memories surface and risk disclosure both to herself and to me. The "treatment" I had provided was tincture of time and a caring and safe relationship. I believe that I did the right thing by not imposing my timeline or trying to prove how smart a doctor I was. In a way, C. G.'s disclosure was her gift to me, her way of saying, "It's working. Keep doing what you're doing." She taught me to be patient, to trust my intuition, and to value who I am as a therapeutic instrument.

Unresolved Grief

Walter W. Rosser
Toronto, Ontario

One of the first patients I encountered, after moving to Toronto, Canada's largest city, was a rather sad sixty-nine-year-old woman who claimed to have been married for more than thirty years. She lived with her husband in a modest apartment on the twenty-ninth floor of one of the twenty-five apartment buildings accommodating more than twenty thousand people in a two-block area of the city. The couple had no children and her husband was moderately disabled from chronic obstructive pulmonary disease.

She told me how she had suffered for thirty-five years from recurrent episodes of abdominal distension accompanied by low back pain. Both of these problems had been extensively investigated by a number of physicians, none of whom had provided a diagnosis or any effective treatment.

I decided to take up the challenge and advised the woman to make visits, even on short notice, whenever her problems were at their worst. This she did over a period of several months. On occasion her abdominal distension was so severe she had to wear maternity clothing. During these periods she had to urinate more frequently and had to modify her posture to that of late pregnancy, which of course further aggravated her back pain. The sight of a seventy-year-old woman looking forty weeks pregnant created considerable anxiety. I was concerned about possible recurrent bowel obstruction, a tumor, or a peritoneal effusion (fluid in her abdominal cavity).

I carefully examined her on several of these occasions and found no physical signs other than the abdominal distension. Concern compelled me to react in a traditional way and order a variety of blood and radiological tests. The test results were completely normal. You can imagine my predicament: the patient was miserable and medical science, as represented by me, was not helping.

I attempted to deal with my anxiety by developing a theory. I hypothesized that her retroverted (tilted) uterus was recurrently trapping and obstructing her bowel, and her condition was aggravated by air swallowing that she would develop at the first signs of discomfort. A gynecology consultant correctly dismissed this theory but offered no explanation for her dramatic symptoms.

A year of follow-up, testing, and consultation passed and no progress had been made in either diagnosing or managing her problem. I continued to work with her and I assume that my persistence in seeking the cause of her problem elicited her trust, because she began to confide in me about a tragic past. She began to hint about a first marriage.

On a day when I was forty-five minutes late, having dealt with a number of administrative and minor medical crises in my office, she opened her heart to the almost intolerable pain of her abusive first marriage. The physical injuries inflicted upon her and her children (she had never previously mentioned a pregnancy) by her first husband were such that she felt obligated to give up for adoption her five children, all under the age of eight, as the best way to ensure their survival. She insightfully wondered if there was any connection between her symptoms and this almost unthinkable event.

Pseudocyesis—false pregnancy—was something I only vaguely remembered from medical school, twenty-seven years ago, but had never seen or considered since. Search of the literature revealed no physiological explanations for pseudocyesis. However, the depth of her pain and unresolved grief provided for me the best explanation of the disturbing and debilitating symptoms that had recurred ever since this tragic event.

During the three years since her dramatic revelation, a program of increased exercise through daily swimming, forty milligrams per day of Prozac, an antidepressant, and occasional office visits for support with the loss and grief she still suffers has resulted in diminished back pain and no further episodes of abdominal distension. The sadness is still there, but it also seems to be diminished.

Epilogue

This experience greatly reinforced the value of two principles of family medicine: continuity of care and the long-term physician–patient relationship. Unfortunately, I have twice violated them through transfers motivated by my pursuit of an academic career.

Cancer, Lies, and Pathology Reports

Mory Summer
Dayton, Ohio

"You didn't hear this one."

About thirty years ago Ghita, my wife, started to have some abdominal pain and cramping. She went to her gynecologist, a friend of mine, who examined her. He felt a fibroid on her uterus and told her that this was the source of her problem and that it had to "come out." No tests, no X-rays, no differential diagnosis; he was "sure."

So a few days later he scheduled her for the surgery. While she was in the operating room, I paced outside. After a long while, the gynecologist came out and told me, "Look Mory, your wife didn't have a fibroid; I opened her up and found a tumor near the cecum" (the first part of the large bowel). Although I was shocked, I somehow had the peace of mind to remember that a general surgeon I trusted was operating at the same time in an adjoining surgical suite. I put on scrubs and interrupted his operation to tell him that my wife was next door on the table with a newly discovered cecal mass. I asked if he could go help the gynecologist and remove the tumor. To free him up I offered to join the assisting surgeon in finishing up his case. He acquiesced and went in to take care of my wife as we finished up his surgery.

My wife is a worrier, and at this time our daughter was one and a half, our son was three, and her father had died of cancer. I felt, right or wrong, that she would be very worried if she thought she had a tumor, that she wouldn't be able to hack it. We sent the mass to the best pathologist around, Ackerman in St. Louis, the writer of a well-known textbook. He wrote back that although the diagnosis of a tumor of the colon (reticulum cell sarcoma) was correct, we were very lucky because it looked like the surgeon had removed the whole thing, and nothing was left, and the margins were clear. No further treatment seemed necessary.

Naturally this is not the end of the story. Ghita worked in my office and had many friends in the hospital and could get hold of her own record. I spoke to a pathologist friend of mine and asked him to write up a fake report on official hospital paper. He went along with the plan and typed up a separate pathology report that noted "inflammatory changes." I brought the report to my wife and said, "See, it was a fibroma, the gynecologist was right."

This ruse lasted for many years and my wife was not troubled by her bout with cancer. However, about twenty years later we were applying for new insurance and a nurse came by to examine us and take a health history. When Ghita stepped out of the room, I told the nurse the real truth about my wife's history of cancer. As you would have it, she walked back in at that moment and heard it all. . . . She didn't speak to me for three months.

References

Balint, M., and E. Balint. 1973. *Six Minutes for the Patient.* London: Tavistock.

Baur, S. 1995. *Confiding: A Psychotherapist and Her Patient Search for Stories to Live By.* New York: Harper Perennial, pp. 54–64.

Burnum, J. F. 1991. Secrets about patients. *New England Journal of Medicine* 324(16):1130–33.

Engel, G. L. 1977. The need for a new medical model: a challenge for biomedicine. *Science* 196:129–36.

GIVIO (Interdisciplinary Group for Cancer Care Evaluation, Italy). 1986. What doctors tell patients with breast cancer about diagnosis and treatment: findings from a study in general hospitals. *British Journal of Cancer* 54:319–26.

Good, M. J. D. 1990. American oncology and the discourse on hope. *Culture, Medicine and Psychiatry* 14:59–79.

Imber-Black, E. 1993. *Secrets in Families and Family Therapy.* New York: Norton.

Kahana, E., D. E. Biegel, and M. L. Wykle (eds.). 1994. *Family Caregiving across the Lifespan.* London: Sage Publications.

McDaniel, S. H., J. Hepworth, and W. J. Doherty. 1992. *Medical Family Therapy.* New York: Basic Books.

Mears, R. 1976. The secret. *Psychiatry* 39(3):258–65.

Medalie, J. H. 1975. The hidden patient. Presentation to the Case Western Reserve University School of Medicine Faculty, Quail Hollow, Ohio, December.

Medalie, J. H. 1994. The Caregiver as the Hidden Patient: Challenges for Medical Practice. In E. Kahana, D. E. Biegel, and M. L. Wykle (eds.). *Family Caregiving across the Lifespan.* London: Sage Publications, pp. 312–30.

Munakata, T. 1986. Japanese Attitudes toward Mental Illness and Mental Health Care. In T. Lebra and W. Lebra (eds.). *Japanese Culture and Behavior.* Honolulu: University of Hawaii Press.

Pellegrino, E. D. 1996. Secrets of the couch and the grave. *Cambridge Quarterly of Healthcare Ethics* 5(2):189–203.

Quill, T. E. 1989. Recognizing and adjusting to barriers in doctor–patient communication. *Annals of Internal Medicine* 111:51–57.

Stewart, M., J. B. Brown, W. Wayne Weston, I. R. McWhinney, C. L. McWilliam, and T. R. Freeman. 1995. *Patient Centered Medicine.* Thousand Oaks, Calif.: Sage Publications.

Toombs, S. K. 1992. *The Meaning of Illness.* Boston: Kluwer Academic Press.

Illness in the Doctor's Family

Reflections

Jon O. Neher

Thanks to illness, the physician's family eats. Day after day, the breadwinner goes to the office or clinic, puts on a white coat (or other culturally appropriate symbol of medical expertise), and cares for the sick. When the day is done, the clinic closed, and all the hospitalized patients tucked in for the night, the physician returns to the seeming security of home and family. Illness, however, will not always be left behind at work.

Disease and disability will visit the physician's home just as surely as it visits every home. When it does, physicians are forced to squarely confront— perhaps for the first time—those scourges they merely brush shoulders with at work. From earaches to problem pregnancies, from Alzheimer's dementia to congestive heart failure, disease is no longer a concept but an experience. The havoc that an illness may wreak upon an individual life and upon the lives of others becomes painfully obvious.

Physicians are naturally tempted to try to help ailing family members with their professional skills. But there are many potential pitfalls in this course of action, particularly around such issues as patient autonomy, confidentiality, physician objectivity, and interpersonal conflict (La Puma and Priest 1992). Wary of these dangers, some physicians completely separate themselves from the doctor role where family is concerned and focus all of their energies on their familial obligations. Others, out of some personal need to maintain control over people or events, cling to the doctor role with raging tenacity, to the detriment of all concerned (McSherry 1988; Freeman 1991). One suspects, however, that most physicians honestly struggle to hold a middle ground where their skills can legitimately contribute to the family during its time of crisis.

Worldwide, most illnesses are mild and are cared for entirely within the family. According to one U.S. study (Boiko, Schuman, and Rust 1984), the home therapies provided by physicians for their family members were surprisingly similar to those provided in the homes of other educated professionals. In fact, lawyers gave their family members prescription medications just as often as physicians did. Physicians were, however, more likely to try to suture small lacerations. In another study (La Puma et al. 1991), 83 percent of 465 physicians practicing at a community hospital in the United States had prescribed medications for family members and 72 percent had examined family members. Somewhat more surprisingly, 15 percent had attended on family members in the hospital, and 13 percent had actually operated on family members. In addition, 33 percent reported observing another physician "inappropriately involved" in the care of a family member and nearly half reported turning down requests for care from family members.

When writing about illness in their families, physician-authors will address three major themes. The first is the primary struggle of the patient with the disease. It is not essential that a physician-author be a family member to write on this theme; physicians tell stories about people with diseases all the time. It is a standard part of their work and is well reflected in the other chapters of this book. However, it is the close family relationship that allows these authors to tell their particular stories in such detail and with great empathy (see "Birth, Death, and Music" and "Uncommon Courage"). Elements of the cultural milieu are frequently described as a literary mechanism to help the reader more fully understand the humanity of the patient.

Alteration of relationships within the family is a second theme in these stories. Illness, in ways both subtle and obvious, removes its victim from his or her usual place within the family and stresses other family members who must cope with the change. Families commonly look to their physician members for strength and guidance, yet physicians may be no more prepared to assume greater responsibility than anyone else (see "Scars"). Familial roles are deeply cultural, and the struggles of family members to compensate for the illness of a loved one are likely to both reaffirm and challenge cherished beliefs. One also suspects that grief from a loss in the family is frequently a motive for writing these narratives.

A third theme is the physician's internal struggle to maintain psychological balance in the face of uncontrollable events. This struggle for equilibrium may be described explicitly in a story or may lend a pervasive tone or texture to the writing (see "You Be the Husband and Let Me Be the Doctor"). As already noted, the one unique option available to the physician is a retreat into the physician role, with its promise of power and control over the elements of disease that threaten the physician's emotional world. Others, however, find peace of mind by attempting to completely recant their physician role (see "Confessions from the Heart"). However balance is found, its realization provides an intimate look into the character of the author.

These three primary struggles—the patient against the illness, the family against change and loss, and the physician against the fear within—are foundational to all stories about illness in the doctor's family. Each story blends these themes in a different way, uniquely illuminating the disease, the individuals involved, the family structure, and the overarching culture. We are allowed to see through the eyes of people who happen to be physicians as they watch their own kin struggle with disease. They have seen the same struggle in patients before and they will see it in patients again. But this time around, they must live intimately with it and its outcome. This time around, disease provides not bread for the table, but the hard kernel of a story.

Uncommon Courage

Howard F. Stein
Oklahoma City, Oklahoma

A decade after the death of my mother, my father remained in the same apartment that had been their home for forty-five years. He asked nothing more than to die in this place where every piece of furniture and window was steeped in memory. His wife, buried in a Jewish cemetery ten miles over the Allegheny Mountains in western Pennsylvania, was this many hills and that many sharp turns up the road to the north. He had visited her grave at least twice a year and driven the same roads for decades before to honor the dead from his synagogue. Many old relatives and friends had died at home while sitting on the toilet. He thought he would prefer this way as well. He had his remaining family well convinced that memories and half a lifetime of familiar surroundings were enough. He wanted no more and he wanted to be nowhere else.

Earlier in his life, he had walked every Sunday morning ten miles through the country. He had inspired neighbors in his declining factory town to walk, long before the medical center touted "wellness" and "cardiovascular fitness." More recently, his walking had become drastically restricted. He did well if he could do his grocery shopping and banking downtown, where most of life's necessities were only a few blocks from home. In warm weather, he enjoyed sitting and sunning his legs on the steps of the Veterans of Foreign Wars service club two blocks from his apartment.

Over the last year, this man was seen out on the streets less and less. Eventually, he could no longer stand and wait in either the heat or the cold to catch the two buses that brought him the thirty miles to his synagogue in Pittsburgh. His daily rounds had shrunk to his apartment and its hallway that circled from the kitchen back to the living room.

Who knows how the years take their toll? Had he too often lifted his sickly wife from her bed and wheelchair? Had isolation and malnourishment been the price he had paid for the constancy of place? All devotions—occupational, familial, religious—exact their cost as they offer comfort. His story is now in his fragile, unbuffered bones. He accepted his circumstances with patience and grace and was grateful to awaken each morning. His supports were a cane; a local hospital's Meals on Wheels; a devoted twice-a-month housekeeper who, except when it snowed, took his dirty laundry to wash at her home; and a man who adopted him as a father and even shopped for his favorite whiskey ("to stimulate his appetite"). For a short while, they sustained the fragile web of his independence.

In mid-November, he fell—no one knows exactly how. A friend had helped him acquire a LifeLine electronic device, one he knew he was to wear all the time yet carefully draped over the bedpost each night. Why, he asked, should he wear it while in bed? He could simply reach for it. Luckily, LifeLine is designed with just such reasoning in mind. When he had not checked in by 8 A.M., the LifeLine operator summoned the police, who had to break into the apartment to get him. Several days of hospitalization for his fractured pelvis, followed by two weeks of visiting nurses' visits to his apartment, could not restore him to independent living. One day, a visitor from his synagogue— a frequent bearer of treasured Jewish breads and pastries—found him unable to get out of bed.

I had thought he was ready to die, or nearly so. And so did he—at least until the long moment when he sat alone in a pool of once-warm excrement. He understood then that death might arrive, but not quickly and not without humiliation. He had outlived by years most of his relatives and friends. To the few who remained, he had held steadfastly that his next and final move would be to the cemetery plot next to his wife, not to any nursing home or any relative's spare room. The granite stone was already bought and in place; all that remained were his name and date of death to be inscribed, as were his wife's.

We say "he changed his mind," but I realize now how little I know about such change or even about him. He is almost ninety; I am about to turn fifty. He is, according to current market value, "unproductive," while I am at least in the wage-earning work force. He, who can scarcely hear even shouting, can tell stories of having heard young Jascha Heifetz and Fritz Kreisler in the 1920s and 1930s, reminding a willing listener what musicality is really about. He, who can scarcely see through his cataracts, still carefully studies biblical and liturgical texts with his "spyglass," as he calls his five-inch-diameter magnifying glass. From his bed, he thinks he still might learn something new. His nursing home clergy are delighted to have more work for themselves, and the rabbi's wife looks forward to bringing him by wheelchair to daily services.

According to the intake worker, who deals with admission requests, when asked about such things as "codes" and "life support," this man nearing ninety said with the same clenched, resolute fist I remember seeing when I was four or five: "I want to live!" He had replied without a second's thought.

He gave up his apartment—his half-century life geography—for his strange and repudiated land, The Nursing Home. At the turn of the century, his parents had fled Romania for the American promised land. I don't know who traveled farther or faced greater uncertainty. My father knew only that when his eldest sister refused a nursing home twenty years ago, the remaining family nearly collapsed under the strain of her care. He did not want this to happen again.

While I stood at his bedside in the nursing home last December, the synagogue friend who had driven him there from his apartment came into the room to visit. "Did your father tell you he wouldn't let us carry him down the twenty-four hallway steps to the car?"

"No," I said, waiting for the rest.

"He didn't want to be carried out. He insisted on going down on his feet. With the aid of three men and his walker, he walked down those stairs to the street one last time."

We both had tears in our eyes as he finished. And, no, my father had not told me.

Confessions from the Heart

Walter L. Larimore and Katherine Lee Larimore
Kissimmee, Florida

In my daughter Kate's seventeen years, she's called me her dada, daddy, dad, father, and friend. In addition, I've been her teacher, physician, and at times, spiritual leader. Of these roles, I have had the most difficulty separating my responsibilities of being her dad from my role of being a doctor. After all, I trained for years for the latter, and the qualifications and training for the former are, as we all know, surprisingly low. Scripture teaches, however, that the responsibility for the role of dad is very high and the results last for generations.

When Kate was born, I was convinced (like most fathers) that she was the most beautiful baby in the history of the world. Even though she was four weeks early and weighed less than six pounds, our first child appeared perfect. But by the time Kate was five months old, my wife, Barb, and I knew something was wrong. By six months a CT scan showed that she had no right brain—just water—and less than 50 percent of a normal left brain. "Just take her home and love her," said the pediatric neurologist. "She will probably never walk or talk." Yet with prayer, love, and therapy she did both—by three years of age.

Five tendon surgeries when she was six and a grand-mal seizure when she was ten kept me humbled, broken, and on my knees. As a family practitioner, I was not able to be her physician for these diseases, and as a human, I could not heal them. This furnace of suffering taught me to trust others, to be served by them, and to cast my anxiety on the Lord (and not reel it back in, as was my habit). But since being a physician was easier for me than being a dad, I was often tempted to follow the more easily traveled trail, even though with Kate I knew I was called to stay on the more difficult road of fatherhood.

After struggling for ten years with my inner doctor–dad conflict, I finally resolved to stay on the dad path and leave the doctor path to my partner, John Hartman. But one Sunday, not long after I made my decision, the temptation "to doctor" instead of "to dad" overcame me.

When Kate turned eleven, we started to go on dates at least once a month. My father had recommended that the first female born into the Larimore family in over eighty years needed some special time alone with her dad—and on a regular basis. During one of those afternoons while we were listening to the radio, I didn't know it, but Kate had something on her mind and needed her dad to listen. Kate said, "Dad, I've been noticing a funny heartbeat again."

She knew this would cause me great concern because she had a very fast heartbeat and felt dizzy and nauseated before her seizure the year before. Instantly, I changed my tone and demeanor. I was no longer in my father mind-set; I was instantly "doctor dad." I felt justified, especially since my partner was out of town and Kate obviously needed to see someone fast.

I was scared. Watching my daughter experience a grand-mal seizure that lasted nearly three hours, required four drugs to stop, and resulted in twelve hours of coma with fixed and dilated pupils—not knowing whether she was brain dead or just deeply sedated—was an encounter I did not want to repeat. I hurriedly asked Kate, "Have you missed any of your medicine? Has Dr. John checked your blood level recently? Any recent fever or colds?"

The only answer that came from my questioning was that episodes always seemed to occur while Kate was at church. "When during church?" I asked almost frantically.

Kate was scared as she tried to think. Then she replied, "Well, it really only happens during my Sunday school class."

I quizzed Kate about the lighting, her activity level, and the tempera-ture in the room, to see if there might have been any factors to provoke a "preseizure aura." [1] But Kate grew tired of my questions—because she knew something I didn't. She wasn't trying to tell me bad news or medically related symptoms. She wanted to communicate the symptoms of her heart. When she'd had enough, Kate put an end to my questions and my compulsive doc-toring by finishing her side of the story.

She said slowly, "Dad, there's one thing that brings on the funny heart-beat in Sunday school."

"What is it?" I asked solicitously.

She continued, "My heart only seems to beat funny when Paul stands up to pray."

When I realized that the symptoms were not of aura but of first puppy love, I felt a simultaneous release of emotion—first relief and then panic. Indeed, the teenage years had begun. So, after drying tears from my eyes, I apologized to my daughter for switching to my doctor hat before using my father ears and heart. I was ashamed at my behavior, because instead of listen-ing, I had taken the easy road once again. Kate was gracious and forgave me—which is more than I can say for myself. Afterward we had a wonderful discus-sion of the attraction that God gives to a woman and a man and how this gift can be used to His glory or misused to our detriment.

That afternoon is still a warm memory, and I'm very thankful for the spe-cial lessons I learned from it. Kate is now seventeen, and I know the Lord will continue to use her to teach me many more valuable lessons as we travel down this path toward the next stage of our lives and our relationship. Today I'm very happy that I made the choice to be Kate's father rather than her doctor. I can't imagine all of the things I would have missed out on had I chosen the easy path.

---

1. An aura is the peculiar sensations, whether visual, auditory, sensory, or vertiginous, felt by patients immediately preceding an epileptic fit.

Birth, Death, and Music

Mats Falk

Alstermo, Sweden

Many years ago, doing my very first locum as a general practitioner, I found myself in an isolated forest community in Småland in the south of Sweden— a community that I was never able to forget and to which I later returned. I now sit here in my old solo practice in the heart of Småland's "Kingdom of Crystal," surrounded by deep forest and a thousand lakes.

The people here, who make a world-famous glass, take pride in their tradition of skilled craftsmanship. However, the use of their lips and lungs is not limited to the glassblower's pipe—they are also called into service to breathe life into their musical instruments. There is, in fact, a musical tradition here that continues to thrive with banners unfurled and ringing tones. Against this backdrop of forest and craftsmanship consider the story of a little human being who was so loved that a specially composed piece of music was dedicated to him, by his father, as a christening present. But the piece was to be played only twice—at the christening and the funeral.

One cold winter's day with a vast sky and a scent of snow in the air, a young man came to me suffering from stomach pains. He was a tall, callow youth with a mass of blond curls; at the age of twenty-one, he already had planted deep roots in the community. I happened to know that he was on his way to a violin soloist examination at the music conservatory.

But now he was ill. It did not take long to discover the source of his problems. With no income and an uncertain future as a professional musician, he was about to become a father. After an intense and passionate relationship, his girlfriend, despite all precautions, had become pregnant. If that wasn't enough, she was expecting triplets. In one fell swoop, he was about to become the father of three!

The mother-to-be, who was small and somewhat frail, had a difficult pregnancy with a lot of pain and a great deal of worry. But each day was a small victory along the road to childbirth. Confined to her bed, she battled against time and pain. In the end, the onset of toxemia[2] hastened the already planned caesarean section.

Finally, the deathly pale father, surrounded by nine green-clad doctors, was able to witness his children's entry into the world with wide-eyed wonder.

A note from the author: Many thanks to Peter Stemberg, who translated the story into English for me.

2. Toxemia is a dangerous metabolic disease of pregnancy marked by high blood pressure, swelling, edema, and other changes.

191

Thirty-four weeks of nervous uncertainty were finally over. The new father of three boys beamed with happiness and paternal pride.

The first two to arrive into the world were Birk and Nathanael. The last was little Jonathan, who was reluctantly weaned from the hold of his mother's womb. It was as if he wanted to stay in the warmth and security of the womb just a little longer. Perhaps it was at that point that he suffered minor brain damage with a slight left-side weakness that revealed itself more clearly some eight months later.

From the very beginning, the little trio of brothers caused a stir wherever they went. Whenever they appeared, they were met by warm smiles and tremendous joy. The triplets' pram alone was a sensation. The christening, which took place in the white village church, was a celebration to be remembered— a local high point with tears of joy and fine music. I was an amateur cellist and I had the privilege of contributing to the celebrations as part of an ad hoc string ensemble, playing a cheerful Haydn quartet. The musical triumph of the day was the duet for violin and cello that the proud father had composed for his three small sons—"The Dance of Triplets." Best of all, I liked the last movement, "Jonathan," a spirited dance full of paternal humility.

Jonathan proved to have inherited his father's musicality. At the age of four, he could recognize and differentiate between the violin concerti of Sibelius, Mozart, and Brahms that his father often played for him. Young Jonathan even developed a preference for Brahms!

One oppressively hot and humid late summer day with a sky full of menacingly dark thunderclouds, I received an extremely worrying report from the young family. Jonathan's condition had suddenly worsened. From having been "best in his class" at the rehabilitation center, he suddenly started to deteriorate. However, the parents felt that their concerns went unheard at the big, impersonal hospital. No one seemed to be able, or have the time, to cope with their worries for Jonathan.

In their desperation, they decided to consult me, their childhood country doctor, remote from all the wonders of modern medicine at the university hospital. Sadly, after a single look, I was able to confirm that the situation was far from positive. Jonathan had developed neurological symptoms on his right side as well as his left. He now had an unmistakable right side ataxia (trouble with coordination) and tremor.

A horrifying thought struck me—brain tumor! I went cold and very nearly lost control of the situation. The full investigative testing machinery was set in motion and a few short weeks later my worst fears were confirmed. Jonathan had a large, completely inoperable, tumor in the pons cerebri, the "bridge" of the brain. After a dangerous and problem-filled neurosurgery, the tissue type was determined—a malignant astrocytoma, a rapidly growing brain tumor.

There followed a terrible period of gnawing worry, desperation, uncertainty, and debilitating radiation treatment. We clung desperately to the faint hope of cure and improvement. But the MRI (magnetic resonance imager), the "oracle" of our time, passed its irrevocable judgment—the tumor was growing apace. The radiation treatment had failed.

Painful uncertainty was replaced by the deepest sorrow. It was quite clear that Jonathan was going to die of his tumor. There was no hope left.

By nature, Jonathan was a gentle, warmhearted, humorous little boy with a passion for food. Toward the end, he drew a great deal of comfort from his humor. The few things that could raise a smile on his pale, deathly serious little face, apart from his pa, were Mr. Bean on video and the visits of the hospital clown. Despite a debilitating paralysis, he was still able to stir his computer games into a rapid frenzy of bleeping, clicking activity. Until the very end, his intellect was always intact.

With childish logic and clear-sightedness during the month-long radiation treatment at the children's oncology clinic, he seemed to have worked out that the difference between life and death was somehow connected to the insertion or noninsertion of the gastric tube. This terrified him. He developed an intense fear of the gastric tube. For Jonathan, it was the messenger of death—oncology's very own private road to Calvary. But a gastric tube had to be employed. No condemned man before his executioner could ever have felt greater fear than Jonathan, faced with the dreaded gastric tube. Without morphine, it would not have been possible. He began to dimly come to the realization that he would never be well again.

For a four year old, death is naturally rather obscure and difficult to comprehend. Even so, it was an ever-present threat of separation and lonesome darkness.

The family talked openly about death. Jonathan knew that he would be going to a star in the sky—but which one? How would he be able to find his way to the right star? He had himself seen the night sky filled with thousands of stars. While he was still able to talk, he had an idea. He wanted to fly to the stars in an airplane himself and check it out. One beautiful day he took to the air, accompanied by his impressive brothers, and returned, visibly satisfied. He had reconnoitered his forthcoming route and seemed to be satisfied with what he had found under his outstretched wings.

As each day passed, the tumor became larger and Jonathan's condition worse. Through nature's own pitiless garroting process he was transformed into an almost blind, speechless, and totally paralyzed wheelchair patient. All the time, with the hateful gastric tube in his nose.

Almost daily, he broke into bitter tears of frustration when no one understood what he wanted or what he meant. With almost imperceptible movements of his eyes, he tried to "point" at pictures and symbols in his meager picture books. For Jonathan, who had just mastered the unique human ability to communicate via language, the loss of this ability to speak was probably the bitterest blow of all. He had to take many unanswered questions with him to his grave.

Strangely enough, the ones who dealt with this crisis best of all were his two brothers. On the advice of the psychologist and thanks to the courage and common sense of their parents, they had been allowed almost total participation and physical access. It was clearly the right medicine. Here, there were no whispering voices or closed doors. Everyone knew that Jonathan was going to die at home.

One Sunday morning in June, while the heavens were filled with birdsong, Jonathan finally took his last breath.

When I joined the family a few hours later, I was met at the door by a friendly smile on the face of Birk. He calmly welcomed me with the words, "Jonathan's dead now—come and see for yourself." And there he lay, almost as transparent and white as an alabaster statue, on his back, in his parents double bed. The pained facial expression had completely disappeared, replaced by an inward, secretive smile. He had been able to die in peace and in the security of the loving closeness of his mother and father.

Birk climbed nimbly onto the bed, put his mouth close to Jonathan's ear, and shouted with all his might: "Jonathan! Jonathan!" When there was no reply, he turned to me and said: "You see, he's dead. He doesn't answer when I call for him."

The other brother, Nathanael, tickled the soles of his dead brother's naked feet. There was still no reaction and he wisely pronounced: "Yes, he really is dead. He doesn't laugh."

Very unusually for Sweden, the funeral began with an open coffin. Everyone felt it a comfort to see him sleeping peacefully in his favorite green striped shirt. His two brothers had, without being aware of it, reconnected the ceremony to one of mankind's oldest burial rituals and furnished him with a number of useful objects for his forthcoming journey to that faraway star. In his arms he held his favorite pillow—his "comforter." At his side lay some of the best toy cars and a jigsaw puzzle inside its little red box, just to pass the time. In his hand he held, unlike the Viking chieftains of old, neither sword nor spear, but a diskette of his best-loved computer games.

And so, for the second time in my life, I heard the "Jonathan" movement of "The Dance of Triplets." But this time it was not tears of joy, but tears of sorrow that coursed down my cheeks. And so ends this story from my long life as a doctor, a story that has affected me more than any other, a story that has changed my life.

Finally, a personal admission—little Jonathan was not just my patient, he was also my beloved grandson.

"You Be the Husband and Let Me Be the Doctor"

Michael Klein

Vancouver, British Columbia

My wife Bonnie is in the intensive care unit, quadriplegic, on a respirator, and "locked in." Her nasoduodenal tube[3] repeatedly becomes dislodged either by accident or because she unconsciously pulls it out. Many hours go by while I wait with her to have it reinserted. The longer she waits, the more fluids, calories, and medications she won't receive by that route. Staff workers are busy; the hospital is short-staffed; reinsertion is a low priority. Some of the house staff are not very skilled at the task and they inadvertently cause my wife great distress. What do I do: Let them practice until they get it right? Merely wait until someone has the time? No, at times I slip it in myself. Some nursing staff are scandalized; others encourage it and are pleased. Some house staff think I am a lunatic; others ask to be taught.

Bonnie is slipping into respiratory failure. It's the weekend. I am alone with a first-year family medicine resident who is cross-covering the neurology service and is doing his best with her and me. Bonnie's neurologist has left for vacation. The covering neurologist from a nearby hospital never comes in to see the patient. I need sleep yet I am sleepless; I have no energy. I am giving up, certain that I will lose her. The resident perseveres and, working with his attending physician, mobilizes the various subspecialist staff who are brought in to consult. Many think that she is going to die anyhow—though each hypothesizes from a different cause. One neurologist thinks that she has a fulminant, malignant, destructive lesion that is migrating in the brain stem. Another neurologist thinks that it is a rapidly destructive form of multiple sclerosis and recommends a cytotoxic drug,[4] which is given. The immunologist thinks that it is a severe form of autoimmune vasculitis[5] and recommends plasmapheresis[6] and high-dose steroids, which are given.

Consultants are postulating multiple and concurrent illnesses. For me, this violates everything I have ever been taught. I can't understand why it cannot be, as originally thought by Bonnie's now vacationing neurologist, a bleed in the brain stem, a diagnosis that would tie it all together. The magnetic resonance imaging that would have settled the matter is not rec-

3. A nasoduodenal tube, a feeding tube made of plastic, is inserted through the nose and passed into the esophagus, stomach, and small intestine.
4. Cytotoxic drugs are medications that are destructive to cells.
5. Autoimmune vasculitis is a disease in which the body's own immune system attacks its blood vessels, causing inflammation and blockage.
6. Plasmapheresis is a process in which blood is removed from the body, separated into its elements, and returned in a plasma substitute.

ommended by the neuroradiologist. The MRI is a scarce resource, and the rationale is that it would be pointless to determine exactly the hypothesized location since it is surgically unapproachable. I am looking for a single fixable lesion and push for the MRI. My specialist colleagues feel that I am over-involved and unrealistic. They reluctantly agree to the MRI, probably to get me off their backs.

We are about to take the ambulance to another center for the MRI exam. I ask the ambulance attendant which method he will use to suction the tracheostomy.[7] He states that he has an electric vacuum suction device.

I ask, "What happens if it fails?"

His reply is self-assured: "It never fails."

Being the suspicious type that I am and a firm believer in the many versions of Murphy's law, I ask for a slight delay while I run up to the delivery suite to obtain a few DeLee oral suction traps.[8] I refuse to be dependent on machines while my wife requires regular tracheostomy suction in order to live. On the trip to the MRI the suction machine fails. I manually suction her airway with the DeLees until arrival at the hospital.

We are about to enter the MRI chamber. The technician says that the test cannot be done. The respiratory technician who came with us, for reasons I do not understand, has returned to our hospital. I think she thought that the MRI center would supply respiratory support. I am bagging[9] my wife by hand while local politics are sorted out. The MRI technician states that the patient is moving too much and ventilation by bag and mask cannot be done during an MRI, because the metal parts cannot be present within the magnetic field. Fortunately, Bonnie needs only intermittent ventilatory support, as she is able to breathe shallowly on her own through the tracheostomy tube. I implore him to let me ventilate between MRI cycles, while he stabilizes her from the other end of the tube. Reluctantly he agrees. Holding her steady for one and a half hours, the technician obtains an acceptable study and is pleased with his efforts despite being so stiff from the ordeal that he can hardly stand.

The MRI clearly demonstrates the lesion. I am alone, staring at the view box, awaiting transport back to our hospital. Although I am an amateur, the lesion looks like it is vascular but encapsulated and benign. The problem is the close placement to the brain stem. Consensus is that the lesion is inoperable. My logic differs. What's to lose? Bonnie is dying and will likely have another bleed. It appears that she has already had two. The transport arrives and I am lost in thought.

Later that day, I organize the transport of multiple MRI copies to neurological friends and colleagues around North America. In a short period of time, they help locate a surgeon in another Canadian city who is prepared to

7. A tracheostomy is an opening, surgically made, into the trachea (windpipe) to assist breathing.

8. A DeLee is a small suction device that works like a straw with a collecting cup.

9. Bagging is the use of a flexible rubber bag (an Ambu bag) to induce artificial breathing.

operate, having been practicing on dogs and awaiting the appearance of the right patient. I am told that no surgeon has been that low in the brain stem before. Patients usually die a respiratory death before the surgeons get to them. Bonnie, still on a respirator, is flown by air ambulance. Even though there is space on the aircraft, I am prohibited from accompanying her and assisting with her care. "It is not done," I am told. I follow with my daughter many hours later on a commercial jet, not knowing if Bonnie is still alive.

Bonnie is in the ICU on a respirator and her tracheostomy needs frequent suctioning. To do this, the respirator needs to be disconnected and she needs to be bagged by hand while the cleaning takes place. I am comfortable with the equipment. Nurse 1 asks me to leave, saying that she cannot do her work with me present. Nurses 2 and 3 integrate me into the care, but there is never a question of who is in charge; they are. Some nurses recognize that working with me not only makes their job easier but is actually "treatment" for me. As long as I feel that I am contributing to the care, I am psychologically better off and more capable of providing support for my wife.

Successful lifesaving surgery is accomplished, removing a huge brain stem malformation that has bled several times. The delicate surgery has wiped out most of one side of the medulla and part of the pons, destroying the nuclei of cranial nerves 9, 10, 11, and 12 on one side: Bonnie can't swallow and one vocal cord is paralyzed. In any case, she can't talk due to her tracheostomy. I am able to communicate with her by a letterboard and a complex system of eye blinks and eventually lip reading. Some of the staff want to learn how to communicate with her, some don't.

Bonnie is having panic attacks and feels like she can't breathe. Some doctors and nurses think that she is "spoiled." "What's her problem?" they say, "we saved her life." Some nurses can partially talk her down from the attacks. Others not only can't but don't want to. They think I am indulging her by gently slowing down her breathing with reassurance and empathy for her paralyzed and powerless state. The normative patient, recovering from an organ transplant or other major lifesaving surgery, is on heavy doses of morphine and benzodiazapine tranquilizers. When they wake up and start getting demanding, they are shipped out for someone else to deal with.

One nurse, equally comfortable with the technical side of the job, wants to learn how to manage panic attacks. There is excellent one-to-one nursing and some nurses are comfortable both caring for Bonnie and dealing with me. I wonder why those who are not comfortable with her and me should be forced to provide care. I work with the charge nurse to create a roster of nurses who want to do the job.

I suggest a pharmacological approach to the panic attacks. The anesthesia staff who run the ICU are uncomfortable with this approach and ask for a psychiatry consult for Bonnie (or for me; I'll never know). The psychiatrist honestly acknowledges that he has not been in an ICU since medical school asks me what I would do. I propose the same benzodiazapine–antidepressant combination that I would use in an office setting. Together we discuss the approach with the ICU staff and a plan is organized. It helps. The nurses who want to care for Bonnie ask me to give them a session on panic attacks. We organize it with the charge nurse. The standard of care dramatically improves and the nurses take pride in their accomplishment.

Bonnie is hospitalized for six months in three different hospitals. I continue to become involved in attempting to improve suboptimal care, and the medical and nursing staff continues to vary in response. Gratitude and a team spirit alternates with anger and harsh words.

So what ultimately is the problem? Anyone who has worked in an institution knows that mistakes are inevitable and happen frequently. People and machines are fallible; in the end we need all the help we can get. Patients ultimately benefit when family members are integrated into their care. Family members contribute valuable information that needs to be weighed, taken seriously, and placed in context. And family members who happen to be health care professionals cannot be expected to disregard all their prior knowledge when planning the course of care for a loved one.

I think the real problem here is fear. It is a fear that we as professionals will be found to be not quite on top of the case. It is difficult for some to say, "I don't know," and to be seen as less than omniscient. Perhaps diagnostic and therapeutic ambiguity, while a normal part of medical practice life, is more difficult to acknowledge to a co-professional who is emotionally tied to the patient. But while I acknowledge that I have a responsibility to express my concerns in the most helpful way possible, ultimately I am much more concerned about Bonnie's health than the feelings of the professional staff. How can one be vigilant but not overbearing? When you figure it out, let me know.

Scars

Michael Malus

Fort Collins, Northwest Territories

"Raynaud's going to get you," Zeno said, shaking his forefinger at me emphatically. Zeno, one of Fort Collins's local traders, had an outsider's clarity
of vision and a streetfighter's acumen. "I've seen doctors come and go. When
Raynaud does not like a doctor," he paused and then whispered, "they don't
last very long!" His forefinger and thumb went from pointing to me to twirl-
ing his mustache, and then became part of a fist that pounded gently but
emphatically on the store counter in front of him. "He's furious about your
trying to block moving the hospital to the new town," Zeno continued. "He
knows you spoke to the chief about organizing opposition."

"So what if he knows?" I asked.

"So what?" Zeno was incredulous. "I can't believe you're that naive! He
wants the new town, right?"

"Right."

"And you're against the new town, right?"

"Right."

"So it's simple. He's going to turn all the people of the town against
you—and get you out of here. He's already started. He's been making points
against you on the death of that kid in Edmonton. You left with the kid, and
the kid came back dead. Then there's those two old guys who died in the first
few weeks you came—Michel Trapper and Samuel Erasmus."

"They were 95 percent dead the first day I got here, they—"

"You don't have to waste your time telling me about it. Of course I know
that. But that's only two of us. And I'm a nonperson here; despised for making an honest living. That leaves you. And how long have you been here? A
year? And how long has Raynaud been here? Twenty-five years. And he speaks
to them in Dogrib with all the sneaky power that someone's own language
can have on them. And he has the fear of hell on his side. You can strut around
with your stethoscope and order airplanes every ten minutes, but all you can
do about a trip to hell is delay it. They believe that in the end whether they
go there or not depends on the balance in their account with Raynaud."

I left the light of Zeno's Restaurant and Pool Hall to enter the dark, sub-
arctic Fort Collins night. Walking home, I thought about the two old men
who had died. They were both permanent residents of the hospital. Michel
Trapper was so old the features of his face were barely discernible in the maze
of his wrinkles. With the Dogrib nursing assistants translating, I used to talk
with him when I was making rounds in the hospital. Particularly on Sundays
when there was no clinic and rounds in the hospital were very relaxed, I had

listened to stories he told of the old ways of living and hunting. He had a tumor of the bladder, which had been operated on several times, leaving him with a permanent urinary catheter. His wife had died many years ago. His children, who lived in distant settlements, would visit him at Christmas and Easter when the whole tribe gathered in Fort Collins. He died one night in his sleep, probably of a heart attack. In other words he just died. His time ran out.

The second man, Samuel Erasmus, had an inoperable cancer of the lung, which spread to his liver and brain. It would have been cruel as well as futile to send him to the hospital in Yellowknife. He passed those last few days among his family and the people he knew, instead of in some strange and terrifying place. The night he died was my first exposure to the Dogrib people's way of dealing with death. Even though he was comatose and didn't hear a thing they were saying, his family and friends came to his bedside and, placing their hands on his in turn, rendered long, wailing accounts of Samuel's virtues as husband, father, and tribal member. They told tales of his prowess as a hunter. They told stories of his knowledge of the wilderness, and his strength and courage in dealing with it at all times. The moment he died they began the arduous task of digging a grave in the frozen ground. It took a dozen men a whole day of digging in the permafrost, in forty below zero cold, to dig a hole deep enough for a coffin.

Father Raynaud was telling the people I should have sent him to Yellowknife. He knows better than that. But as Zeno says, the truth is not the issue here. I am in Raynaud's way. That bastard! Blaming me for the deaths of those old men! And for Lawrence Arrowmaker's death!

I felt really low. But not as low as the day I sent my own four-month-old son Allen out with severe dehydration from gastroenteritis[10] that proved near fatal. I sent Allen to the University Hospital in Edmonton, a thousand miles south of us. A nurse went with him to regulate the intravenous fluid he was receiving in flight, and my wife, Lenore, went as the one-parent escort government regulations allow. To this day Lenore gets angry and can't really look at me when she remembers how I sent them out alone and didn't go with them.

She's absolutely right. Of course I should have gone with them. I was stupid. I made the decision thinking as the doctor at Fort Collins and not as a father and husband. My reasoning at the time was based on the fact that the government paid for one parent to accompany a child as an escort. I could have paid for myself, but I felt that as the doctor in the settlement, I would never again be able to face parents in the same situation who couldn't afford to do what I could. Also, I was going to be superfluous in Allen's medical care. In retrospect I could have asked for coverage of Fort Collins from doctors in Yellowknife, as I learned was possible several months later, when I took

---

10. Gastroenteritis is stomach and intestinal inflammation.

Lawrence Arrowmaker, the baby who died in surgery, down to Edmonton. Beyond all these theoretical considerations, the net result was that for very superficial reasons, I sent Lenore with Allen a thousand miles away to fight for his life in an unknown hospital in a strange city. Every time I think of it I cringe at my stupidity and callousness.

On top of everything else, I had made a mistake in Allen's treatment, which was a major factor in the severity of his dehydration. At one point, when he seemed to be getting slightly better, one of the older nurses suggested giving him clear soup. I knew it was sentimental and a scientifically unsound idea. But I wanted to believe he was better. An hour after eating the soup he began to vomit and have diarrhea again. A doctor at Edmonton told Lenore that the soup had played a role in his subsequent deterioration. Lenore could barely speak about it on the phone.

I pictured for a moment Lenore sitting alone with Allen critically ill—a needle in his scalp for hydration—in a hospital a thousand miles away knowing I was partially responsible for his condition. It was too horrible to contemplate. Allen recovered over the next few days, thank God. Wounds in the body heal by scarring. Marriages have their scars as well. Over the years scars can fade and become less noticeable. But they are scars nonetheless, and the pain they commemorate is nonetheless pain.

Walking home from Zeno's, I thought of that morning when Allen and Lenore were being taken to Edmonton. When I heard the evacuation plane approaching, I ran to the chief maintenance man's house to find out where a runway had been cleared. The site of the runway would sometimes change because of snowdrifts and wind conditions. The chief maintenance man was a white man who was an appointee of the town manager. I had never had any previous dealings with him, but since the town manager and Father Raynaud saw me as a troublemaker, I knew the chief maintenance man would feel the same way.

I could hear the plane approaching. In my haste to find out where the runway was, I stepped into the chief maintenance man's house without taking off my snowboots. He made a big fuss about it. "Didn't you ever learn to take off your snowboots before you come into someone's house?" he snarled derisively.

"You're right. I'm sorry," I answered hastily. "But my kid is critically ill. He's being evacuated. Time's very important here. It's a matter of life and death. I just want to know where the runway's been cleared—"

"But you could have stood outside until I came to the door," the chief maintenance man persisted. The plane engine was sounding louder and closer, and I still didn't know where the runway was. The chief maintenance man continued relentlessly: "You didn't have to come in here with your boots all covered with snow and drip it all over the place!"

I grabbed a broom which was near the door and swept away the small amount of snow my boots had carried in. "Okay? Is that all right now you son of a bitch?!" I yelled. "Now where is the goddamn runway?" I grabbed him by the collar. "If you don't tell me in the next two seconds, I'm going to kill you!"

I was well written up for that episode by the chief maintenance man with my medical superior's help. I was described as displaying behavior not befitting a medical officer. The fact that Allen was critically ill and the maintenance man was withholding vital information was never considered relevant.

When Allen and Lenore were down in the hospital in Edmonton, I had no one to help take care of my four-year-old son, Mark. Once I had to take him with me on a medical trip to a settlement—for which I was duly written up. I was criticized for having a member of my family accompanying me while on medical duty and using public transport for family members.

I was being written up passionately, voluminously, and endlessly for what was essentially a civilian court martial, which would occur when renewal of my contract came up after a year on the job. I was starting to feel weary of constantly being on trial, with no one to speak in my defense except me. It added to the strain of being the only doctor—and a relatively inexperienced one at that. At times I would feel bad about my inexperience. My mistake with Allen, for example.

Lenore had tolerated the isolation and hardship of living in Fort Collins so that I could do the kind of medicine I wanted to do. At some level, too, I was aware that there was no doctor with more experience who wanted to come here and that I was doing the best I could.

But that night as I walked home from Zeno's it was cold and the dogs were howling. Father Raynaud was blaming me for deaths for which I was innocent. I was tempted to knock on Raynaud's door and invite a write-up for which I would be guilty.

References

Boiko, P. E., S. H. Schuman, and P. F. Rust. 1984. Physicians treating their own spouses: relationship of physicians to their own family's health care. *Journal of Family Practice* 18:891–96.

Freeman, D. L. 1991. Heal thyself. *Annals of Internal Medicine* 114:694.

La Puma, J., and E. R. Priest. 1992. Is there a doctor in the house? an analysis of the practice of physicians treating their own family. *Journal of the American Medical Association* 267:1810–12.

La Puma, J., C. B. Stocking, D. La Voie, and C. A. Darling. 1991. When physicians treat members of their own families: practices in a community hospital. *New England Journal of Medicine* 325:1290–94.

McSherry, J. 1988. Long-distance meddling: do MDs really know what's best for their children? *Canadian Medical Association Journal* 193:420–22.

Epilogue

Jeffrey M. Borkan and William L. Miller

What are the benefits of stories in medicine? Medical stories such as those presented in this book are "good" for physicians *personally* and *professionally.* To begin with, as Hunter (1991:xxi) writes, "Understanding medicine as a narrative activity enables us—both physicians and patients—to shift the focus of medicine to the care of what ails the patient and away from the relatively simpler matter of the diagnosis of disease."

Reaching agreement on the story line engenders patient satisfaction, implies caring and support, and maximizes the perceived and objective relief of sickness. It has even been postulated to be the basis of the placebo effect (Brody & Waters 1980; Brody 1987). The success of the negotiation can determine the level of patient adherence to the medical regimen (Greenfield, Borkan, and Yodfat 1987) and influence the prospects for symptom resolution. Several recent studies and a US National Academy of Sciences Institute of Medicine report suggest that illness outcomes, particularly those associated with pain, may depend more on doctor–patient interaction than on diagnostic and therapeutic techniques (Osterweis, Kleinman, and Mechanic 1987; Starfield et al. 1981; Spiegel et al. 1989; Henbest and Stewart 1990). Clinicians take for granted that constructing a good clinical story from the history of the present illness leads to a correct diagnosis and can also be therapeutic (Adler 1997). The therapeutic effect results from the patient "feeling better" and even "healing better" from the experience of narrative formulation (Lehrman 1993; Adler 1997). Just reaching agreement with the patient on the diagnosis may improve outcomes in common primary care problems (Fitzpatrick, Hopkins, and Harvard-Watts 1983; Bass et al. 1986; Headache Study Group 1986). Attaining consensus may require a shared language, something which can be achieved only if the physician empathizes with and attempts to understand his or her patient's experiences. The meaningful and effective application of evidence-based medicine requires the contextual understanding that comes through the patient's story. Only through the story can we access the patient's local knowledge and experience, so important when considering diagnostic or treatment plans. This can vary from the impact of drawing blood from someone for whom this is taboo to suggesting the use of cholesterol-lowering drugs, with their inherent potential for liver damage, in someone whose father died from liver failure.

Medical narratives can be used therapeutically in other ways. Storytelling may give patients, particularly those with chronic, debilitating, or terminal diseases, the opportunity to resolve, rewrite, or rescript conflicts and find both resolutions and proper endings to their autobiographies (White and Epston 1990). It can also rekindle hope: empathetic listening, translation, and interpretation are the craft of the clinician who cares for the chronically ill (Kleinman 1980). After an illness such as stroke, behaviors emerge from personal histories (Kaufman 1989). Should the patient see himself as a "loser" in all things, rehabilitation may be doomed to failure. An intervention might include reviewing the person's life history in order to emphasize previously overlooked or underplayed events, which could provide the source of a new self-image. Each visit, although complete in itself, becomes incorporated as a chapter in the larger story of the person's life. Co-writing the script for the future overcomes barriers to health and may lead to a new sense of coherence. Similarly, when we embrace the metaphors and symbols our patients use (i.e., if we really listen), we can often assist them with insights and/or provide helpful substitutions.

What advantage can the physician derive from listening to patients' stories? In addition to the therapeutic aspects mentioned, paying attention to narratives may have added benefits that are not readily apparent. For instance, seeing our patients, especially the more "difficult" ones, as seasoned storytellers may increase our appreciation of them and improve our enjoyment of clinical medicine. Physicians often complain of the unidirectional flow of energy in clinical sessions. These same doctors may be renewed and reinvigorated if they begin to see their patients as striving to create original, meaningful stories.

Years of listening to the stories of patients can even create new roles. For instance, in many small towns and neighborhoods the physician acts as a kind of "clerk of records" (Berger 1967; Brody 1987), the repository of the stories that give the community its meanings. The doctor does more than treat people when they are ill; he or she is "the objective witness to their lives" (Berger 1967). Over time, the community physician can serve as a point of reference for community knowledge and identity, offering a sense of history and stored wisdom.

On a professional level, the stories in the preceding chapters may be useful as training tools to medical students, residents, and those in the early years of practice. They provide an important humanistic approach to the practice of medicine today—something ever more critical as technology, bureaucracy, and business weigh in to control doctor–patient interactions. In addition, they are useful for those veterans in general and family practice who may need refreshing in order to hear their patients or their own unique stories.

Finally, on a personal level, what is our story as healers? This book has presented many examples. How do we want our story told, heard, and remembered? If we use our own stories as a mirror for who we are and what we pay attention to, perhaps we can co-evolve with our patients, becoming more aware of both their and our own worlds. We hope that the stories presented in this volume will make a difference to the reader by both enriching and increasing understanding of the human condition. Perhaps they can also nurture a new generation of healers and healing stories. This book is not complete, and the stories are not perfect. There is always hope, however. The story is still being written. Do you hear it?

References

Adler, M. 1997. The history of the present illness as treatment: who's listening, and why does it matter? *Journal of the American Board of Family Practice* 10:28–35.

Bass, M. J., C. Buck, L. Turner, G. Dickie, G. Pratt, and C. Robinson. 1986. The physician's actions in the outcome of illness in family practice. *Journal of Family Practice* 23:43–47.

Berger, J. 1867. *A Fortunate Man.* New York: Holt, Rinehart and Winston.

Brody, H. 1987. *Stories of Sickness.* New Haven: Yale University Press.

Brody, H., and D. B. Waters. Diagnosis is treatment. *Journal of Family Practice* 10:445–49.

Fitzpatrick, R. M., A. P. Hopkins, and O. Harvard-Watts. 1983. Social dimensions of healing: a longitudinal study of outcomes of medical management of headaches. *Social Science in Medicine* 17:501–10.

Greenfield, S. F., J. Borkan, and Y. Yodfat. 1987. Health beliefs and hypertension: a case-control study in a Moroccan Jewish community in Israel. *Culture, Medicine and Psychiatry* 11:79–95.

The Headache Study Group of the University of Western Ontario. 1986. Predictors of outcome in headache patients presenting to family physicians: a one year prospective study. *Headache* 26:285–94.

Henbest, R.J., and M. Stewart. 1990. Patient-centredness in the consultation: 2. Does it really make a difference? *Family Practice* 7:28–33.

Herman, J. 1990. Anger in the consultation. *British Journal of General Practice.* May, pp. 176–77.

Hunter, K. M. 1991. *Doctors' Stories: The Narrative Structure of Medical Knowledge.* Princeton, N.J.: Princeton University Press.

Kaufman, S. R. 1988. Stroke rehabilitation and the negotiation of identity. In: S. Reinharz and G. D. Rowles (eds.). *Qualitative Gerontology.* New York: Springer, pp. 82–103.

Kaufman, S. 1993. *The Healer's Tale.* Madison: University of Wisconsin Press.

Kleinman, A. 1980. *Patients and Healers in the Context of Culture.* Berkeley: University of California Press.

Lehrman, N. S. 1993. Pleasure heals: the role of social pleasure—love in its broadest sense—in medical practice. *Archives of Internal Medicine* 153:929–34.

Osterweis, M., A. Kleinman, and D. Mechanic (eds.). 1987. *Pain and Disability: Clinical, Behavioral and Public Policy Perspectives.* Washington, D.C.: National Academy Press.

Spiegel, D., J. R. Bloom, H. C. Kraemer, and E. Gottheil. 1989. Effect of psychosocial treatment on survival of patients with metastatic breast cancer. *Lancet,* pp. 888–91.

Starfield, B., C. Wray, K. Hess, R. Gross, P. S. Birk, and B. C. D'Lugoff. 1981. The influence of patient–practitioner agreement on outcome of care. *American Journal of Public Health* 71 : 127–32.

White, M., and D. Epston. 1990. *Narrative Means to Therapeutic Ends.* New York: Norton.

Contributors

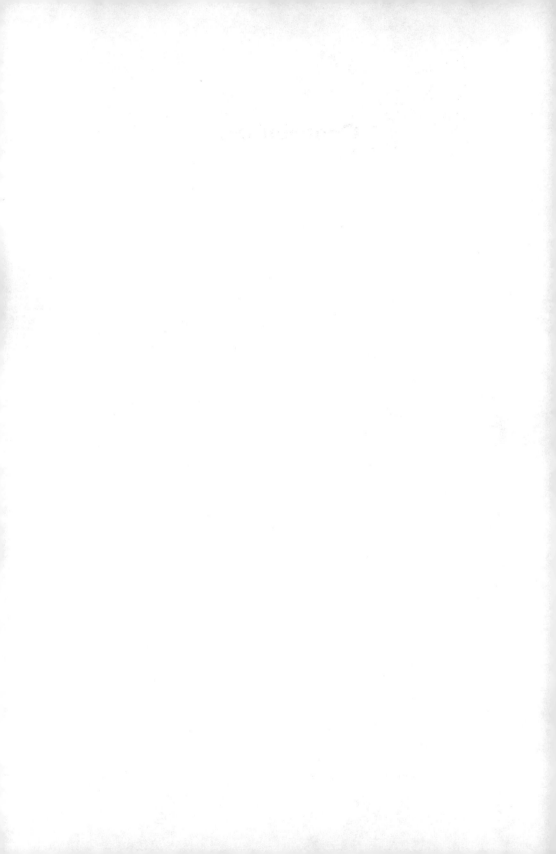

Contributors

This section contains brief biographies of the authors, commentators, and editors.

MARIO AHRENS was born in Argentina in 1933. He is a 1960 graduate of the University of Buenos Aires School of Medicine. For two years, not able to decide on a specialty, he practiced general medicine in the health service of a large oil company in Buenos Aires. In 1963 he moved to the United States to train. While still in training, he became disenchanted with the social and political upheavals of Argentina and decided to stay in the United States. He married Karen, now a clinical psychologist. They have two daughters—plus three children from a previous marriage and five grandchildren. Thirty-two years later, after a career that included active-duty service in the U.S. Navy, he retired to pursue other interests: hiking in the mountains of the Pacific Northwest (from his home outside Seattle), kayaking, painting, and last but not least, writing. When at the end of his clinical practice he put pen to paper, Julio and Venancio presented themselves, demanding their story be told. The story is based on his own experiences, though he admits that forty years may have added the patina of time to the settings and a nostalgic aura to the memories.

JUSTIN ALLEN has been a general practitioner in rural Leicestershire in the heart of England for twenty-five years. Most of that time he has been teaching and running a training program for general practice trainees—the equivalent of a family practice residency. Since 1991 he has been involved with the teaching of general practice in Europe through the Royal College of General Practitioners International Committee and EURACT, the European Academy of Teachers in General Practice. He is also Joint Honorary Secretary of the Joint Committee on Postgraduate Training for General Practice, the U.K. standard-setting body for general practitioner training. In his spare time he sleeps.

HANS ANTONNEAU was born on February 19, 1956, in Leuven, Belgium. He studied medicine at the Catholic University of Leuven, from which he graduated in 1980. Since graduation, he has been in general practice in a group of six in Antwerp. He is on the faculty of the Department of Primary Health Care of the University of Antwerp, where he primarily teaches first-year residents in general practice. In his clinical practice he trains students and vocational trainees (interns and residents). He is father of three girls and a boy. He devotes his free time to being a father and to writing stories, mostly for children. He is also the leader of a professional theater for children.

CSABA ARNOLD was born in 1936. After graduation from medical school, he worked for four years as a solo general practitioner in a rural area. He has been lecturing at the Semmelweis University of Medicine, teaching general practice and family medicine since the early 1970s. Dr. Arnold was appointed the first head of the Department of Family Medicine in Hungary in 1993 at Semmelweis. He is currently continuing as director, as well as practicing part time as a family physician in a rural community.

AYA BIDERMAN, born in Israel in 1953, studied medicine at the Hebrew University in Jerusalem. She decided to enter family medicine, even though it was quite a "new" profession in Israel. She is now the deputy chairperson of the Department of Family Medicine at Ben-Gurion University of the Negev, in Beer-Sheva. She is the medical director of Yud-Aleph Clinic, a large teaching clinic in Beer-Sheva, a southern city in Israel. She also teaches students and residents in family medicine, and her main interests are the physician–patient relationship, communication, and the family in medical care. She is married and has three daughters, two of whom are now in medical school. In her little free time she loves to travel and to hike and has visited many beautiful places around the world.

JEFFREY M. BORKAN divides his professional time between clinical family practice in a remote desert area of southern Israel, research, writing, and teaching. He is director of research in the Department of Family Medicine and lecturer in medical anthropology at Ben-Gurion University of the Negev in Israel. For many years, he coordinated the RAMBAM Israeli Family Practice Research Network, which he helped to found. Prior to moving to Israel, he completed his studies in medical anthropology and medicine at the University of Michigan, Case Western Reserve University, and Harvard University, and he served on the faculty of the University of Massachusetts Medical Center, where he continues as assistant professor. He lives on a kibbutz in the Negev Desert with his wife, Suzanne, a clinical social worker and dairy woman, and their three children, Ariela, Noa, and Aidan. His family is his chief joy, though he also enjoys hiking, running, writing, and singing. He has always been an avid story-listener and storyteller, even constructing a new story every night for his children at bedtime. Putting together this book has been a labor of love—a combination of interests in the humanities and health care, where the tale often "tells it all."

RUTH BRIDGEWATER works part time as a general practitioner in a working-class urban practice. She also teaches and undertakes research. She has a passionate interest in attempting to make storytelling an acceptable mode of medical research. She is on the faculty of the Department of Primary Health Care, University of Newcastle, Newcastle upon Tyne in the United Kingdom.

HOWARD BRODY completed his MD in 1977 while also working on a PhD in philosophy at Michigan State University. He then completed a residency in family practice at the University of Virginia Medical Center. Since returning to Michigan State, he divides his time between the Department of Family Practice and the Center for Ethics and Humanities in the Life Sciences, which he directs. One of his research interests is the role of narrative in both medical practice and medical ethics. He explored these questions in his groundbreaking book, *Stories of Sickness* (Yale University Press, 1987).

KATHY COLE-KELLY, a family therapist, has been teaching family practice residents and medical students the past fifteen years. She is the director of psychosocial education at Metrohealth Medical Center's Department of Family Practice and co-directs the clinical sciences curriculum at Case Western Reserve University School of Medicine, where she is an associate professor. Her areas of academic interest include families and health, families and chronic illness, effective physician–patient communication, class, race, gender, and ethnic considerations. She also has a small private practice in marital and family therapy. In addition to work, Ms. Cole-Kelly loves to *play*, both with friends and with family. She loves to explore the wilderness, where she is at her happiest. When restricted to the city, she runs, bikes, and swims. She is forever grateful for her privilege of working with and learning so much from Jack Medalic.

PETER CURTIS, originally born and trained in England, works as a family doctor, faculty member, and researcher in the Department of Family Medicine at the University of North Carolina, Chapel Hill. He thinks stories and history are vital to our families and our society and regards Robin Hull as a fine mentor and a wonderful writer.

GEORGE L. ENGEL is Professor Emeritus of Medicine and Psychiatry at the University of Rochester, New York. For fifty years his work has ranged over the fields of medicine, psychiatry, psychoanalysis, and psychosomatic medicine. He has more than three hundred publications in eighty different journals, forty textbooks, and symposia on a wide range of topics. His landmark article in *Science* on the biopsychosocial model has been cited more than a thousand times since it appeared in 1977.

MATS FALK has been practicing general medicine almost twenty-five years at the Alstermo Primary Health Care Center, a small solo practice in the "Kingdom of Crystal," where the famous hand-made Swedish glass is still produced. He has devoted his life to his remote practice, hidden in the forests of Småland in the south of Sweden, deeply concerned about the doctor–patient relationship. Dr. Falk thinks that this relationship is the most important tool in clinical practice. To him the art in the "art of medicine" is to try to improve this tool constantly, in a process of lifelong learning. This is best achieved at a solo practice, with its almost complete continuity and accessibility. He has published a humorous book, *Doctor Owl at the Forest Clinic*, with 148 anecdotes and cartoons from his long life of "unforgettable" consultations. Apart from being a writer, he is also a musician, playing the cello, a composer, writing small pieces of chamber music, and a well-known speaker, preferably talking about his main interest: how to build and utilize the doctor–patient relationship in clinical practice.

PERLE FELDMAN was born and raised in Montreal. She demonstrated her first interest in childbirth at age eight, when she performed a forceps delivery on a guppy. She attended McGill University, receiving an undergraduate degree in psychology and a medical degree there. After a confused and checkered postgraduate career, which included a rotating internship and time in obstetrics and pathology residencies, she became a family doctor. She has a strong interest in maternal and child health. Her best and most important ongoing work is her family, which includes her husband of twenty-one years, David Glaser, and their four children, Alison, Erica, Emma, and Josh.

SHIMON GLICK is an American by birth, an internist-endocrinologist by medical training. He moved to Israel in 1974 with the opening of the Ben-Gurion University Medical School, where he was the first chairman of the Department of Internal Medicine and subsequently the dean. He currently is professor of medicine at the school, and he heads the Center for Medical Education. He also teaches medical ethics at the school and is on Israel's national committee for the regulation of human experimentation. He has recently assumed the post of ombudsman for Israel's Ministry of Health. He is the father of six and the grandfather of thirty-three.

FRANCES GRIFFITHS is a general practitioner in an industrial town in northeast England. She has been in practice for ten years. She has also researched women's attitudes to hormone replacement therapy and holds a doctorate in sociology.

JOHN C. GUNZBURG has been a general practitioner since the early seventies and is now devoting his time to psychotherapy. He published extensively in the *Australian Family Physician* and is author of two books, including *The Family Counselling Casebook* (McGraw-Hill, 1981). He is married to Joy and is the father of three daughters.

CAROL P. HERBERT is professor and head of the Department of Family Practice at the University of British Columbia in Vancouver and editor of an international journal, *Patient Education and Counseling.* She was the founding head of the Division of Behavioural Medicine in the Department of Family Practice. Her current research interests are in clinical health promotion and communication in primary care. She is leader of the Family Physician Study Group of the BC Research Satellite Centre of the National Sociobehavioural Cancer Research Network, which is engaged in a number of studies regarding decision making and communication. She has recently completed a participatory research project on diabetes education, with the Haida community and community physicians in the Queen Charlotte Islands. She has been a leader nationally and internationally in the development of primary care research, and she is a past chair of the National Research Committee of the College of Family Physicians of Canada and a past president of the North American Primary Care Research Group. She is current chair of the National College of Family Physicians of Canada Committee on Child and Adolescent Health. Dr. Herbert is a fellow of the College of Family Physicians of Canada and is the winner of the 1997 W. Victor Johnston Medal for lifetime contribution to the College of Family Physicians of Canada.

JUDITH HOLLIS-TRIANTAFILLOU is a British-trained medical practitioner who has lived for many years in Athens, Greece, working in the fields of primary health care and research. She is a founder member of SEXTANT Company, a multidisciplinary research and consultancy organization, and has a particular interest in the social aspects of health.

BENEDIKT P. HORN was born in 1942. He has been in general practice for twenty-one years in Interlaken, Switzerland. He is married to Irene, also a physician, and they have four children—none of whom have entered medicine! He is professor for general medicine at the University of Berne. His hobbies are music, theater, opera, alpinism, gardening, and being a "house-man."

DOMINIQUE HUAS is currently the vice president of the National College of Teaching General Practitioners and a national representative to the European General Practice Research Workshop. He practices clinical medicine in Paris, France, where he lives with his wife (also a general practitioner) and family.

ROBIN HULL, now living in Scotland, is a retired professor of general practice and president of the General Practitioners Writers Association, whose journal he edits. He has published some five hundred articles on a wide variety of medical and allied subjects from alcohol to zoonosis. He has written several books on general practice and palliative care and worked on thirty educational television programs. He has lectured internationally and has published crossword puzzles in four journals.

KAMI KANDOLA is currently completing a two-year residency program in international health at Johns Hopkins University in Baltimore, Maryland, as well as a masters in public health. She recently returned from working in a mission hospital in primary and community health care on the Ivory Coast of West Africa.

MICHAEL KLEIN is a family doctor, a fellow of the College of Family Physicians of Canada, and head of family practice at BC Women's and Children's in Vancouver, British Columbia. His wife, Bonnie Sherr Klein, is an award-winning filmmaker and writer whose book *Slow Dance: A Story of Stroke, Love and Disability,* based on their experiences, was published by Knopf Canada in January 1997. Despite her stroke, Bonnie functions autonomously and continues to improve nine years after the aneurysm burst.

ARTHUR KLEINMAN is one of the most influential scholars in medical anthropology and social medicine today. He is the Maude and Lillian Presley Professor of Medical Anthropology, professor of Psychiatry, and chairman, Department of Social Medicine, Harvard Medical School, and professor of Social Anthropology, Department of Anthropology, Faculty of Arts and Sciences, Harvard University. He has conducted cross-cultural research since 1968 on illness experience and health care in Chinese society and in North America. More recently, he has studied political violence, other forms of social suffering, and their moral and policy implications. His research career began with ethnographic studies of local health care systems in Taiwan, China, and the United States. From this vantage point he organized an anthropological framework for studying illness experience, help seeking, clinical communication, the work of doctoring, and the culture of biomedicine. Then he turned to cross-cultural comparisons of depression, somatization, the social course of chronic medical illness. More recently his research has widened to encompass the broader domain of suffering as sociosomatic experience that links together moral, political, and psychophysiological conditions such as violence, trauma, and social breakdown. Professor Kleinman is the author of more than 150 articles, author of five books, editor or co-editor of fifteen volumes, and the founder of the journal *Culture, Medicine and Psychiatry.* He lives with his wife and co-researcher of many years, Joan Kleinman, in Cambridge, Massachusetts.

WALTER L. LARIMORE is in a small group family practice in Kissimmee, Florida. He provides a wide range of family practice services including maternity care, sports medicine, and geriatric care and procedures. His greatest privilege is being best friend to his wife of twenty-three years, Barbara, and a parent and friend of Katherine L. Larimore and Scott B. Larimore. However, he considers his most vital relationship the one he has with his Father in Heaven, the Great Physician.

ROBERT C. LIKE is an associate professor of family medicine at the University of Medicine and Dentistry of New Jersey–Robert Wood Johnson Medical School in New Brunswick. He is a practicing family physician with a background in family health science, medical anthropology, and health services research. He has carried out fieldwork in the Azores Islands, Portugal; Beersheba, Israel; Zuni, New Mexico; and the Kingdom of Tonga in Western Polynesia. He is especially interested in multicultural education and the delivery of family-centered primary health care to vulnerable populations. He is married, has a four-year old son, and enjoys reading, classical music, swimming, and trying to make the world a better place.

ANN C. MACAULAY graduated from medical school in Scotland and immigrated to Canada in 1969. In 1970 she was hired by a First Nations community near Montreal to help in the development of their new community-controlled health services and continues to work there as a family physician. In the early 1980s she became interested in the very high rates of diabetes and its complications in First Nations. Today her position includes participatory research with this Mohawk community for the primary prevention of diabetes. Dr. Macaulay is also an associate professor in family medicine at McGill University, where she enjoys the challenge of teaching family medicine residents and medical students in the multicultural city of Montreal. Her interests include tennis, cross-country skiing, music, reading, and exploring the world through conferences and, more important, by visiting her two children, currently working in South Africa and Hong Kong.

MICHAEL MALUS is chief of the Department of Family Medicine at the Sir Mortimer B. Davis Jewish General Hospital of the Herzl Family Practice Center in Montreal, Canada, and an associate professor of family medicine and pediatrics at McGill University. He has a special interest in adolescent and Native health. He has worked in rural settings and native communities in Canada and the United States.

JACK H. MEDALIE's life experience and career have been rich and varied. Though born and currently living in the United States, he spent most of his life in South Africa and Israel, serving both in World War II and in the Israeli War of Independence. He received his BSc and MD degrees from the University of Witwatersrand, South Africa, where he earned "colors" for football all four years. As a postgraduate, he received his MPH (cum laude) from Harvard School of Public Health. With four others, he founded, developed, and lived on a cooperative farming settlement, Moshav Habonim (1949–1953), in Israel. After this he became the medical director of Hadassah Family and Community Health Center, Jerusalem, Israel, and professor and chairman of the Department of Family Medicine, Tel-Aviv University. In 1975, he was invited to Cleveland, Ohio, to found and develop the first Department of Family Medicine in the School of Medicine, Case Western Reserve University. Before he retired as chair in 1987, he founded and developed residency programs with clinical departments at five local hospitals and developed and directed the Robert Wood Johnson Foundation Family Medicine Fellowship Program. During his career he has received many awards, including a Fulbright Fellowship, election to the Institute of Medicine of the National Academy of Sciences, and Honorary Lifetime Fellow of the American Academy on Physician and Patient. He has written two books and is currently preparing a third one, has written seven methodological research manuals, and has contributed twenty-six chapters to books edited by others and 129 articles to peer-reviewed medical journals. He is currently semiretired, though continuing as professor emeritus at Case Western Reserve University and seeing patients three days a week.

THOMAS M. METTEE is currently an associate professor at Case Western Reserve University School of Medicine, in addition to having his own family practice clinic in Chesterland, Ohio. He served for many years as the director of the family practice residency at Metro Hospital in Cleveland and was active in community-oriented primary care.

WILLIAM L. MILLER is a physician-anthropologist at Lehigh Valley Hospital in Allentown, Pennsylvania, where he is vice-chair and program director of a newly formed family medicine residency program. He has been active in an effort to make qualitative research more accessible to health care clinicians and researchers. He has contributed book chapters and articles detailing step-by-step applications of qualitative methods, including the book *Doing Qualitative Research,* which he co-edited with Benjamin Crabtree. His research interests center on the role of the patient–physician relationship in health care, on physician and patient understanding of pain, and on hypertension.

JON O. NEHER is the assistant director for education at the Valley Medical Center Family Practice Residency in Renton, Washington. He is also a clinical associate professor of family medicine at the University of Washington, Seattle. He has published a variety of plays, doctor stories, editorials, original research, and light verse. He loves hiking and the outdoors.

IVAR OSTERGAARD graduated from medical school in Denmark in 1973. He has worked as a family physician since 1978 and became a specialist in family practice in 1980. Since 1982 he has been a family medicine trainer and since 1986, associate professor of family medicine at Aarhus University. He is a member and a chair of various national and international task forces and committees on education and educational research. He has contributed scientific papers on various topics relevant to clinical family medicine, with a special emphasis on palliative care. He is currently the secretary of the EURACT (European Academy of Teachers in General Practice) board.

WILLIAM R. PHILLIPS is a private practice family doctor in Seattle, Washington. His university degree was in creative writing and he is devoted to understanding his patients and their stories. He earned his MD and his MPH at the University of Washington and is residency trained and board certified in both family practice and preventive medicine. Dr. Phillips is clinical professor of family medicine at the University of Washington and has worked in Australia, New Zealand, and Zimbabwe, in addition to Seattle. He is active in teaching and research and is the recent past president of the North American Primary Care Research Network.

C. J. ALBERT RATULANGIE was born in Bandoenag, a town in West Java, Indonesia, where his mother was a doctor—one of the first Eurasian women to enter medicine. She inspired, but in no way prompted him to enter medicine. He studied at the University of Amsterdam and qualified as a physician in 1952. Currently he is a general practitioner in Spain, where he moved with his family in 1985. Previously he worked in Africa for ten years (Ghana, Nigeria, and Tanzania) and later he was a general practitioner in Curaçao, West Indies. In his current solo practice in Spain, most of his patients are expatriates, though he has Spanish patients as well. His office is only about 400 meters from his residence in La Nucia, in a small coastal town between Alicante and Valencia. The town is on Spain's Costa Blanca (White Coast)—a very popular region among tourists, old-age pensioners, and the young from all over western Europe. His favorite pastimes are tennis and golf. In the evenings he and his wife like to play bridge or chess with friends. Further spheres of interest are the history of medicine and anthropology.

SHMUEL REIS is a family physician, currently the chairperson of the Department of Family Medicine, a department that is striving to combine "high touch" (humanistic practice) with "high tech" (evidence-based medicine), in Haifa, Israel. He combines patient care in the rural western Galilee with teaching and research. Dr. Reis is presently working on a masters degree in health professions education in Maastricht, The Netherlands. He has served the same patient population for approximately twenty years. He is a founder of a unique family practice center which provides integrated health and social services in a collaborative fashion. He teaches and mentors extensively at a variety of levels, from students to seasoned practitioners. Major research topics include low back pain and the assessment of competence among medical students and physicians. He is a student of professional and personal development of physicians, patient-doctor communication, and the social responsibility of doctors. He is married to Noa, father of six, and ready, though not expecting soon, to become a grandfather. Working on this book was a "peak eperience" where mind and heart and more were involved and nurtured.

WALTER W. ROSSER graduated from Queen's University in Kingston, Ontario, in 1967 and completed three years postgraduate training in family medicine. Currently he is the professor and chair of the Department of Family and Community Medicine at the University of Toronto. He previously served terms as the chair of family medicine at both McMaster University and the University of Ottawa. An active researcher, Dr. Rosser has published extensively in peer-reviewed national and international primary care journals and is the co-author of two books, the most recent entitled *Evidence-Based Family Medicine* (1998).

MINDY SMITH, from Chelsea, Michigan, is an associate professor in the Department of Family Practice at the College of Human Medicine, Michigan State University. In this role her activities include patient care, teaching in the department's family practice residency program, and for the medical school, research and writing. Dr. Smith received her MD degree from the University of Michigan Medical School in 1980 and completed a Family Practice Residency Program at Southern Illinois University in 1983. She was awarded a masters degree in research design and data analysis from the University of Michigan, School of Public Health in 1986. Dr. Smith has published extensively in the area of perinatal care, and she served as guest editor and contributing author for a 1993 issue of *Primary Care on Obstetrics*. She is also an associate editor for the journal *Family Medicine*. She is married and the mother of a four-year-old daughter. The family enjoys travel throughout the United States and Canada, where they may be found soaking in hot springs, hiking mountain trails, or collecting rocks. She is a part-time gardener and carpenter's helper.

STANLEY G. SMITH graduated from Trinity College, Dublin, in 1960. After a period of internship in Ireland and England and a trainee assistantship in general practice in London, England, he moved to Canada. After fourteen years of private practice in Regina, Saskatchewan, Dr. Smith joined the College of Medicine, University of Saskatchewan, to be the residency training director of the newly established program in family medicine. Dr. Smith went on to become the chair of the department, a position he held until recently. He is now a faculty member of the Department of Family Medicine at the University of Western Ontario.

KURT C. STANGE is a practicing family physician, teacher, and epidemiologist. He is associate professor of family medicine, epidemiology and biostatistics, and sociology at Case Western Reserve University, where he is also the Cancer Center associate director for prevention and control and a Robert Wood Johnson Generalist Physician Faculty Scholar. Dr. Stange lives in the Cleveland, Ohio, area with his wife and two children.

HOWARD F. STEIN, a medical anthropologist, psychoanalytic anthropologist, organizational anthropologist, organizational consultant, political psychologist, and psychohistorian, is professor of family and preventive medicine in the Department of Family and Preventive Medicine at the University of Oklahoma Health Sciences Center, Oklahoma City and Enid, at which he has taught for twenty-one years. He directs the behavioral medicine curriculum at the Enid Family Medicine Clinic, the rural-based family practice residency program in northwest Oklahoma. Although he presents lectures, seminars, and workshops to interns, residents, and medical and physician assistant students on a myriad of topics, he feels he is most clinically useful in individual resident and faculty consultations, in listening to trainee and patients' stories, in visiting with nonphysician staff to learn the medical organization's story(-ies), and in "hanging out" around the nurses' station and in the clinic hallways, awaiting an unanticipatable "teaching moment." He is more process-oriented than "expert" in content. In the last fifteen years he has led nearly a thousand Balint groups for interns, residents, faculty, and community physicians. He is author, co-author, or editor of twenty books and more than two hundred scholarly/clinical articles and chapters. From 1980 to 1988 he edited *The Journal of Psychoanalytic Anthropology*. In 1997 he became president-elect of the High Plains Society for Applied Anthropology. He has been an active member of the Society of Teachers of Family Medicine since 1980 and has been a frequent plenary speaker at the Hinsdale Forum for the Behavioral Sciences in Family Medicine series held annually in the Chicago area.

DOV STEINMETZ is a practicing family physician in three rural kibbutzim in northern Israel. He has an academic appointment as a lecturer at the Faculty of Health Sciences, Ben-Gurion University of the Negev, Beer-Sheva. He teaches medicine to residents, mainly emphasizing the psychosocial aspects of medicine. He is a graduate of the Haifa School of Psychotherapy and leads Balint groups. During a year as a visiting scholar at the Ohio State University, Department of Family Medicine, in Columbus, Dr. Steinmetz conducted qualitative research about the way family physicians care for dying patients and their families. He believes the holistic approach is the best way for people to take care of themselves. He has a private clinic where he integrates his knowledge and experience in family medicine, psychotherapy, and complementary medicine, mainly bioresonance therapy and Bach flower remedies, an alternative discipline.

BOB STEVER is a retired family physician in Seattle, Washington, who has lived and worked extensively in troubled areas of Asia. His university degree was earned at Swarthmore College in 1957, and his medical degree is from the University of Pennsylvania. His experience in Asia began with six months of clinical clerkships in north India and Nepal in 1960 and continued with two years in Kratie, Cambodia (1962–1964), and on Quaker medical aid teams to North Vietnam and post–Pol Pot Cambodia. For nearly twenty-five years, he was a family physician at the Health Cooperative of Puget Sound. He has gathered special stories from all of his experiences, including the one in this volume. He is also the author of book of collected stories, entitled *Magic Moments as Paths Cross.*

MORY SUMMER was born in 1929 in Chicago, the son of a custom tailor with no "medical heritage" anywhere in the family. He lived and went to school in the poor area near the Cook County–University of Illinois medical complex. He entered pharmacy school in that complex in 1947 "by serendipity," but he switched to medicine a year later—"the dental, pharmacy and medical school were all in the same building and it seemed that you could do more with your life and your work by being a physician." After completing studies, he did a rotating internship, also at Cook County, and then volunteered for the U.S. Air Force. Expecting to go to some exotic locale, he instead landed in the middle of Kansas at a Strategic Air Command (SAC) bomber base with his new bride, Ghita. In the Air Force he gained broad experience, and instead of returning for an obstetrics residency, decided to continue with general practice. After looking around, he joined a small group practice in Dayton, Ohio, in 1961. Within a few years he became a partner in the practice, continuing after his partners died or retired. In nearly 40 years in practice here, he has cared for nearly two continuous generations of Daytonians—deliveries, surgeries, emergencies, inpatient care, outpatient care. He is planning to retire, glad to finish with some of the changes in medicine—managed care, endless paperwork, and "attitudes." After retirement he will devote time to his hobbies—fishing, weightlifting, bowling, gardening, and cooking, specializing in cakes, jams, and jellies, to expand into breads when possible.

IGOR SVAB was born in 1957 in Ljubljana, Slovenia, and graduated from the Medical Faculty there in 1981. He became a specialist in general practice in 1989 and received his PhD in medicine in 1993 for his work "Multivariate Analysis of the Reasons for Referral from General Practice." He worked in a rural health center from 1983 to 1991, at the beginning as a GP, later as a director of the center. He is currently chair of the Department of Family Medicine at the Medical Faculty and adviser at the Center for the Research of the Health of the Population at the Institute of Public Health. He is also a member of the editorial board of the *European Journal of General Practice*.

HAVA TABENKIN is the chairperson of the Department of Family Medicine for the Northern District and Ha'emek Medical Center in Israel and a senior lecturer at Ben-Gurion University, Faculty of Health Sciences. She works as a family physician in kibbutz clinics in the Jezrael Valley and is also a first-year student in the Law Faculty, Haifa University. She is a veteran member of Kibbutz Ein Harod, is married, and has three children.

MICHAEL WEINGARTEN studied at Oxford and London before moving to Israel, where he was one of the earliest residents in family practice. He is in clinical practice in Rosh Haayin, a town of Yemenite immigrants, and he has described his patient population in *Changing Health and Changing Culture* (Praeger, 1992). He is director of the Department of Family Medicine at the Rabin Medical Center, near Tel-Aviv, which runs the largest Israeli residency program in family medicine. He is also chairman of the Continuing Medical Education Committee of the Israel Medical Association, chairman of the Israel Family Medicine Research Network, and editor of *The Israel Journal of Family Practice*.